Beyond the Barbell

Confessions of a Female Fitness Competitor

NATASHA KOSTALAS

KINGSLEY
PUBLISHERS

First published in South Africa by Kingsley Publishers, 2025
Copyright © Nastasha Kostalas, 2025

The right of Nastasha Kostalas to be identified as author
of this work has been asserted.

Kingsley Publishers
Pretoria,
South Africa
www.kingsleypublishers.com

A catalogue copy of this book will be available from
the National Library of South Africa

Paperback ISBN: 978-0-6398420-3-5
eBook ISBN: 978-0-6398420-2-8

'This book is more than a memoir. Natasha's journey is a true testament of resilience..with raw authenticity and courage, it is a deeply moving and inspirational read' – **Shelli Epstein (Sportsperson and author of 'Flying High: Lessons from the Big Top')**

'Natasha's book demonstrates that the mind can take you places where the body could not alone.' – **The Fit Factory**

'Insightful and emotional, Natasha delves deep into 'aftercare' sor bodybuilding competitors and the highs and lows of a sport so revered.' – **Katieliftz- (Powerlifter, bodybuilder and holds the American Record Bench)**

'For anyone looking to gain a deeper, reflective insight and take away some important lessons...a valuable read!' – **Loz Vickers (Coach and Bodybuilder)**

'An honest view of being on the inside of the fitness world' – **Suni Kanda (Professional Makeup artist of bodybuilding shows)**

'An empowering and candid exploration of the challenges and triumphs women face in the fitness world. A must-read for anyone looking to embrace their own fitness journey with confidence and authenticity.' – **Ashley Ward (Former professional Rugby player and coach)**

'If you've ever chased a body and lost yourself in the process, this will hit hard'- **Palma Szalo (Entrepreneur and bodybuilder)**

'Anyone who reads this will be truly inspired' – **Bilsy Shah (Serial Entrepeuner and former boxer)**

'Valuable and helpful, not only for so many competitors, but for all people wanting to approach the gym' – **Rachel Kiddo (Miami Pro Fitness Model)**

'An amazing insight and detailed perspective of what competing is like for the first time, which included many aspects of life that are less spoken about'- **Zone Gym**

'A powerful look into the hidden struggles behind extreme fitness and the restrict-binge cycle that so impacts competitive athletes...a valuable contribution to awareness and recovery'- **Kathryn Hansen- (Bestselling author of 'Brain Over Binge' and 'The Brain over Binge Recovery Guide')**

'Very informative and inspirational at the same time. As real as it gets.' – **Dr Zak Pallikaros- (Founder and Owner of Pumping Iron Gym)**

'Natasha shares her heart so vulnerably and openly you feel seen and heard by her story'- **Lucy Superfox- (Former presenter of Pure Elite)**

'This is more than a book; it's a reminder of the power we all hold within us to rise above life's challenges'- **Jonathan Kumuteo – (Professional boxer)**

'A raw and powerful exploration of the complex realities of being a female fitness competitor'- **Karl Morris- (Professional fitness photographer)**

'An inspiring story for anyone chasing change' – **Tyrese Johnson-Fisher- (sportsperson)**

'This is a truly remarkable book that will help many understand the complex world of female bodybuilding competitors – **Danielle Spencer- (Makeup Artist and bodybuilding show glam specialist)**

'A brilliant insight into the world of competing...a worthy read for anyone looking to or has delved into the world of female bodybuilding'- **Black Ice Bikinis**

Natasha's story reflects incredible ambition and the courage to see your dreams through' – **Anna Sward, (Author of The Protein Pow cookbook)**

For my brother Anton Kostalas,
who gave me the strength to transform my life.

For my mum.
You instilled in me a love of books and it has shaped who I am today.
I've fulfilled our dream, so this journey is as much yours as it is mine.

To weight training -
you helped me discover who I really am and to
be proud of the person I've become.

Colour key to my own quotes highlighted in the book

S TRESS

T RANSFORMATION

R ESILIENCE

O PTIMISM

N EEDS

G RATITUDE

Contents

Foreword by Anton Kostalas

(BA Hons in Sport Science, Kostalas Coaching)

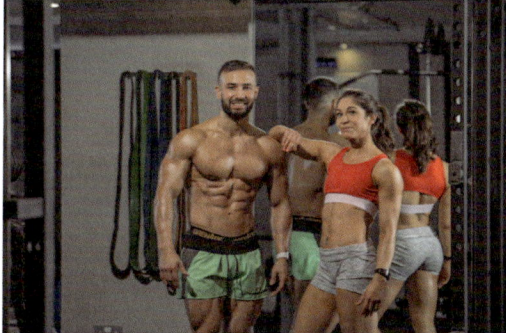

One day, with a thrilled expression on her face, my sister sat me down and announced she was going to write this book. I cannot describe the feelings of pride that enveloped my entire being as she muttered those very words.

I felt proud, not just as her brother and that close bond we share, rare to find in other sibling relationships, but as her coach too. I was so honoured when she asked me to write this foreword, someone who knows her nearly as much as she knows herself and even more honoured to be a part of the next stage of her fitness career.

Fitness meant everything to my sister and I, even when we were growing up. Playing Piggy in the Middle with a ball in our back garden, riding our bikes aimlessly, playing tennis and just getting into mischief, we weren't kids that sat in front of the TV all day, we'd get bored too quickly!

We loved being in the great outdoors, grateful for our dad to have been a school caretaker and so making the most of access to playgrounds, tennis courts and fields. We relished in it, especially during the school holidays. Friends of our parents would often express their shock that we never got bored or irritable in each other's company, we never argued and that still stands today in our thirties.

Fitness still means everything to us, just as much as it did back then.

We were each other's rocks when we went through the most painful time of our lives, our parents' divorce, and we were only teenagers then. But, we had each other and that is all that mattered.

You may know Tash as the ambitious, successful teacher. You may know her through following the growth and development in her fitness journey and across the fitness industry. You may be her close friend, or you might not know her at all. You may have just picked up this book because you are someone who has just started their own fitness journey and has that hunger to know as much as you can about a female's truth and competing.

What I can tell you about my sister is that she speaks the absolute truth about *everything*.

She is the most unique individual you will ever meet. She is raw and real, more so than many in our industry. What you will read in the pages that follow are her own words, her own unique experiences and her truth about competing from a natural female bodybuilder's perspective. What she speaks is heartfelt and delves into so much more than fitness; mental health, depression, hopes, failures, successes, relationships, personal struggles and her rebirth as an individual.

The very beginning of her fitness career long before becoming a Fitness Coach and even before competing, was the rebirth of not just her new life, but who she has become as a person. She has finally found an identity, her own authentic self, where she fits in this world, her ultimate happiness being her goal.

You don't need to be in fitness to relate to her story. Her story is unique but relative to any ordinary person in this world, no matter their background or lifestyle.

My sister had tunnel vision when it came to her teaching career. She started becoming a lot more stressed with marking, staying late at work, and working relentlessly on weekends. I didn't think it was a problem at first, but when she started becoming a lot more negative, abandoning time to eat or even drink during the day and putting work before her own needs, I became concerned.

A few years later, she went through the darkest time in her life, and I felt helpless. She was embarking on a lot of personal issues and depression crept up on her in the most savage way imaginable.

"Tash, you need to start prioritising yourself. When you are ready, just come and train with me twice a week, trust me when I say it will make you feel better." That's all I said to her.

I am unsure how much time had passed, but eventually she agreed to train with me. I was excited because I knew this would be the start of making her feel so much better about herself. I knew learning to lift would make her stronger, both physically and mentally.

A couple of months into training and Tash had become so much stronger and her moods started to improve as well as her sleep. One thing led to another and she made it known that she wanted to learn more. We got her so deep into it, she started learning about calories and how it could help get maximal results in her performance.

After a long period she announced: "Ant, I want to compete."

It seemed her ambitious nature didn't just limit her to teaching. She was finally investing something in herself and putting herself first.

My sister has finally taken that route and she deserves it, because I am sure you will read further in this book, she does not regret any decision she has ever made, no matter how painful or how difficult those decisions.

Fast forward to today and my sister and I are finally working together, something I never dreamed would ever happen in the past. We are building our business in order to help as many men and women as possible transform not only their bodies, but their entire mindsets towards becoming more active and more positive. Learning they can build a healthy, stronger body that can be sustained for the rest of their life.

There are so many people who believe the life they are living now is their life forever, but I am sure that there's something in your mind that you know deep in your heart you have always wanted to accomplish, but you have buried it under responsibility and expectation. My advice; don't bury it, you will never know where it might lead.

Anton Kostalas 2021

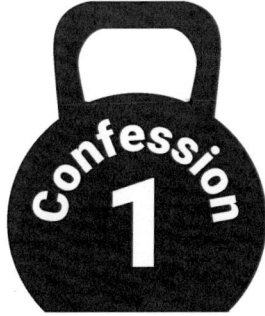

My "Why"

"Either write something worth reading or do something worth writing."
Benjamin Franklin

There is a reason you have purchased this memoir. You may be interested in fitness: you may train religiously; you may train sporadically; you may not even care for training and fitness at all. You may just be curious about the world of someone who is in the fitness industry. You may know me personally, through social media or of me through someone else. You may be a past, current, or even future client. You may not know of me at all. But, regardless of your acquisition, be aware that everything that is written here is the full truth; my own confessions of what it's *really* like to walk in the heels of a Female Fitness Competitor.

Please note that everything has been written in my own words, my own voice. For me, hiring a ghost writer would have eroded the personal journey you and I are on.

If you haven't met me yet, this is most likely the closest thing you will come to doing so. As you traverse the pages of this memoir, the instigation of reflecting on YOU may ensue. You may ponder how active you are in your own life; how much you value your mental and physical wellbeing or whether you too have a deeper calling; a purpose or goal that may not necessarily be related to training at all.

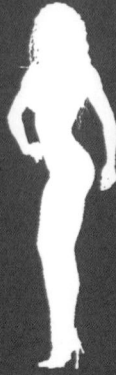

Being inspired always leads to a call of action. Once you have that courage to follow your dream or passion, the end result will phenomenally surprise you.

Alternatively, if what is written here encourages you to start training for your own "why" then it may even persuade you to go down the competing path, or it may adjourn it completely. That is for you to decide. It may teach you so much more about yourself than you may ever come to realise, even if not immediately. It may teach you to be brave. It may present a world of discipline, something already instilled in your life, or something too obscure to ascertain. It may just be a fascinating and insightful read and above everything else, I hope this is how you view it when you reach the end. Something I learnt was how being inspired always leads to a call of action. Once you have that courage to follow your dream or passion, the end result will phenomenally surprise you.

The ultimate reason I decided to write this memoir was the hope to commit to a mental recovery journey that I could share with you all. I knew I needed to rescue myself from the depths of despair and disappointment; to eliminate this mourning behaviour I had adopted; to try and diminish the failure I had felt and regrettably become.

I began writing the week after I formed the painful decision to walk away from the competing world and withdraw from two shows due to my mental health and other personal circumstances precipitating its decline. Although I am someone who wears their heart on their sleeve, writing about my inherent feelings has given me a new goal, motivated me to focus on something different, renewed my passion for writing and bestowed me the ultimate release from everything in my head.

It is shocking to discover the rarity that this topic holds in books of the fitness industry and the unmitigated avoidance of it altogether. Competing in bodybuilding involves much more than making big sacrifices, I can assure you. There is a darker side. It is taboo, and even competing itself holds its own imposter syndrome. Despite listening to podcast episodes and reading handbooks on fat loss and training, I am surprised that no one has really dug deeper than that, to write a book on what it's *really* like to be a fitness competitor, traversing the vicissitudes of the mind.

Beyond the glitter, beyond the glamour, beyond the stage.

I yearn for this memoir to shock you, enlighten you, humour you, inspire you. I want it to make you think about what life means to you and what it's been like for me and also for everyone else in my world at that time. It transpires more than just fitness.

I have had two separate lives; the one before competing and the one after. That is not to say that I have adopted chameleon tendencies, but once you compete, your life really does change forever. You are not a completely different person but an altered one, yet you never forget your previous self. It is the catalyst in reshaping pivotal aspects of your life, whether that is your relationship with food, your relationships with the people closest to you, your habits, and your mindset, all of which alter indefinitely.

Change is a positive thing; without change there is no opportunity for growth. Being inspired, following your passion or dream and having the courage to turn it into an action is ultimate satisfaction, leading you to become inspiring to others.

Before I share my story, it's important for you to understand my competitive background. This background provides the context for the challenges and achievements that have defined my path, has formed my experiences and decisions, shaping who I am today.

At the age of twelve or thirteen, a lingering sense of inadequacy in the early years of secondary school, caused me to conclude that I was not good enough: 'We prefer positive self-evaluations... because they indicate our social worth... they satisfy our desire for communion and interpersonal connectedness with others... the communion motive emphasises people's acceptance and belongingness.' (Swann and Bosson 2010)

Change is a positive thing; without change there is no opportunity for growth.

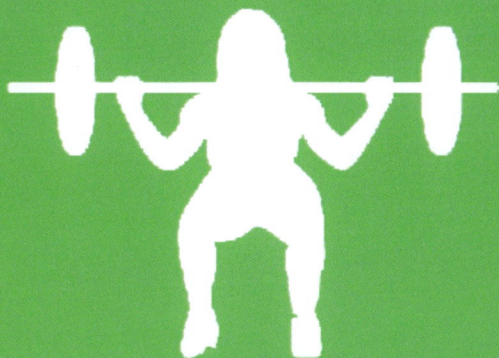

I never really felt pretty enough, skinny enough or popular enough in comparison to my peers. I was never part of the 'popular' group, but I wasn't a part of the "boderick" or "geeky" group either. In the bustling halls of my school, I was the invisible, quiet one. I worked hard, diligently completing everything expected of me, striving for excellence yet only making it into the top set for English, the only place where I truly felt I excelled.

My efforts were often overshadowed by the louder, more confident students around me; I was the goody-two-shoes who found solace relentlessly trying to prove myself and gain praise from my teachers, often, with my head in a book. In my appearance, I was that Greek girl with the thick, frizzy hair, the nerdy one, with heavy framed glasses, the uneven eyebrows, the slightly bent teeth. I was the girl that no one ever fancied. This persistent sense of inadequacy was my first solid opinion about myself; compounded by comparing myself to others who seemed to excel, effortlessly, physically, socially and intellectually.

I was just average, blending in, inconspicuous. Outside of school, I had two hobbies: ballet and playing the piano, both of which I started at age five.

I wasn't amazing at sports although I was in the girls' netball team. However, the only other talent I had was being one of the fastest girls at the 100m sprint in my year group. I remember as far back as primary school where I was always picked first for batting in rounders because everyone knew I'd be the one winning all the home runs.

When I was about twelve or thirteen, I remember competing in the County Athletics My mum sent me to the Queen Elizabeth Stadium (the Athletic Club for Enfield and Haringey). Surrounded by kids who had clearly done the sport for years, made me feel out of place and discouraged, so I convinced my mum not to send me there anymore. The frustration of not measuring up took the fun out of it. I still wonder to this day if I had persevered in athletics how good I could have become. How successful would I have been?

Sports days at the end of the school year was the one day I had the speed to outpace everyone else. Coming in at the back of the group of four relay runners was my moment. A moment where my athletic ability shone. I could hear all my peers yelling my name. Their voices grew louder with every stride, fuelling my determination, filling me with adrenaline, driving me to cross that white line. I loved that thrill and, hands down, it was the only time where I felt huge confidence in myself.

From a young age I'd sit with my dad as he watched the Olympics, captivated by the 100m sprinters. I admired their powerful, chiselled bodies. It was the first time I became aware of appearance and developed an admiration for aesthetics. Valuing their strength and physical excellence, I thought to myself, I wanted to look like them one day. As I watched the slow-motion recap at the end of the races, I was in complete awe of how the competitors' muscles looked and moved. Those moments sparked a lasting impression on how I viewed fitness and my own body goals; the undoubtable beauty of athleticism.

The first time I picked up a fitness magazine in my early teens, I was captivated by the image of a strong, confident woman with ironing-board abs and the title: 'Do 200 sit-ups a day to look like this'. I found myself longing to look and feel like her. In that moment a desire ignited to make it my mission. Every day before school, I would complete one hundred sit ups and the same again before bed. Despite my dedication, I soon became disheartened when I didn't see the changes I had expected; questioning whether my efforts were in vain.

I would spend hours watching MTV staring at idols like Joss Stone and Jojo, performing in trendy crop tops exhibiting their flat tummies, while I would sing along to their songs, comparing myself to their seemingly perfect bodies and growing increasingly critical of my own appearance. And this was at a time before social media and the likes of Instagram!

Although my confidence would heighten and dip throughout my teenage and early adulthood years, hands down, the worst I ever felt about myself was after I had competed in 2019. But shockingly, even on the day of my shows in peak condition, I'd stare at myself in the mirror backstage, focusing on every perceived flaw and imperfection thinking; I'm not lean enough; in that moment I would be transported back, the insecurities of my youth echoing around me.

This constant self-criticism eroded my confidence when my body changed a short while after competing and there were many occasions driving to work where I would tell myself: *I am not worthy to be in the fitness industry.*

This tells you one thing. There are consequences to competing in bodybuilding. Consequences that can create an illusion of flawless health and fitness. You obsessively compare yourself to others, you obsessively compare yourself to your peak condition. Comments years later would often wound me; the look of shock when people discovered what I once was. Looking back on my once "perfect'" body, all along I should have reminded myself that perfection does not exist and that striving for it was unrealistic and unfair to myself. Instead, I should have focused on doing things that made me the best version of myself, embracing my unique strengths and qualities. Shifting my mindset from unattainable ideals to personal growth and self-improvement would have brought me greater satisfaction and happiness.

Who is the real Natasha Kostalas today?

Despite how I may come across on social media in presenting myself, I will always view myself as *ordinary*. But even ordinary people can share fascinating experiences. You may ask, well what is *ordinary?* I guess, I have always viewed myself as an everyday, normal individual you'd pass in the street and possibly not even notice. Yet, my experiences, which I have been so desperate to share, surpass this view of myself.

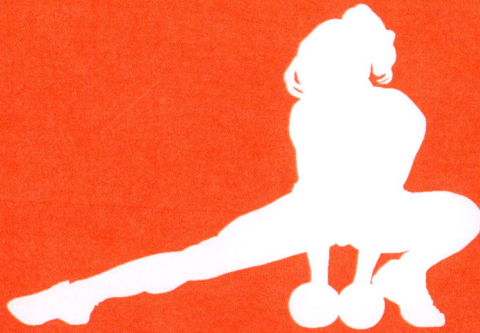

Gratitude has been a big part of my journey. Recognising how far I've come, acknowledging the people and situations which have brought me here.

Reflecting on my life now, with the wealth of knowledge I've gained in relation to competing, I can see how I've embraced both the good and the bad. At times I have laughed, cried, been relieved, been thankful. Gratitude has been a big part of my journey. Recognising how far I've come, acknowledging the people and situations which have brought me here, recognising that I am ultimately responsible for the journey I have taken; for the person I have become and the moment I am living in.

Each confession in this memoir is the *real me* pouring out my heart. I want you to know me without ever meeting me. I want you to embark on the fitness journey I hold before you, feel the feelings I have felt, observe the growth through my trials and tribulations, endure my suffering and behold the happiness of my exultations.

Yes, I wrote this for me, for my own mental therapy but I also wrote this for you. I listened to a podcast once where a successful writer said: 'publishing a book was a business card on steroids.' To be frank, I don't care much if this doesn't become a number 1 bestseller or tops the charts on Amazon or makes it into every book shop window. I don't mind if you dislike it, I wouldn't mind if you relished in it, my only wish is you personify it, and *learn something* from it. Learn something about me the competitor, but something about YOU as an individual.

THANK YOU. I am forever grateful to you for choosing to pick up this book, giving some time of your day to read it, whilst you ponder your thoughts with every turning page.

I confess I truly hope you enjoy it.

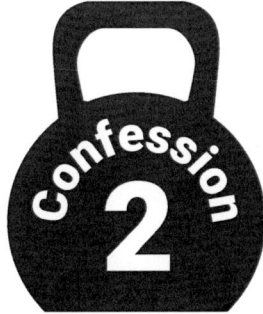

The Magic Moment

"The future depends on what you do today."
Mahatma Gandhi

This is my most interesting and most surprising confession to you; the truth about why I *really* started weight training.

Believe it or not, it was NEVER to compete or even to change my body composition. Honestly, I was so far removed from even thinking about aesthetics, having one hundred and one other things racing around in my head at the time.

Despite the usual insecurities that most females tolerate, the last thing I cared about was my body and how others viewed it, habitually accepting but disregarding the opinions I had of myself and secretly imprisoning them in my mind.

I read once about an interesting concept that psychologists have around identity and how the concept of our selves is bound with how others see us, known as the concept of "looking glass self" (Cooley, 1902) Our self-worth can mirror that of other people's thoughts and feelings: "our self-views form as a result of our perceptions of other people's opinions of us." Hence, on reflection, I remember the misconception I held for a long time about males and females who trained or worked in the fitness industry. I believed that if they shared the aesthetics of individuals on the front of magazines, they were ignominiously boastful of their successes, prone to habitually projecting their arrogance like peacocks spreading their tail feathers and living everyday shamelessly projecting their elitist attitudes.

If anything, this said more about me; someone with incredibly low self-esteem, inadequacy, narrowmindedness, and a complete lack of confidence outside of my teaching career.

To understand the context, we must rewind back to 2015. September 1st to be exact. I had started my prestigious new job as a Head of English at a school in Enfield, North London; a mere four years into my teaching career, a naïve twenty-six-year-old, given an amazing opportunity with a huge role and the weight of the school's GCSE results hanging on my shoulders.

Sauntering assuredly through the main entrance the first day, clutching my handbag filled with various notepads bursting with colour, a new pack of pretty biros and my personalised teacher planner with my name dominating the front cover, I walked in with purpose. The rush of anticipation raced through my veins before I was to meet my new department. Yet, stepping into this daunting hall filled with hundreds of teachers, voices echoing in unison before the INSET (teacher training day) was to commence, a sense of inhibition took over. Expelling any such demons instantly, Little Miss Confident took command and feeling so accomplished, embraced this fear of responsibility, really believing this to be the evolution of success in the profession, the only thing I was ever destined to do, or be.

As a twenty-one-year-old Newly Qualified Teacher in July 2011, I was probed in the interview with that most common question: 'Where do you see yourself in five years?' Without delay, my answer with the utmost assurance: 'A Head of English, of course.' My ambitious nature ensured I achieved it within four.

I was brilliant at my job. Remaining the humble individual I'd always been and still knew I was. Just to give you some understanding of my capabilities, two weeks as a newly qualified teacher in September 2011, I was graded "Good" by Ofsted, having been observed with the most difficult Year 11 class (fifteen and sixteen-year-olds) the whole school had ever known. To receive a "Good" was not what I was expecting; this small class made up of only eleven students was at the time for any new teacher, the class from hell. The students had severe behaviour problems and low literacy levels. One, whose behaviour was so volatile that even anger management classes could not reform him. It was a failure I was expecting. Yet in the end, they had proved to be the most genuine, honest and grateful class I was ever to teach. I may not have reformed them in their characters, but I certainly aided their achievement of grades higher than their predicted ones and I instilled in them a gratitude, I least expected.

A couple of years later, I was observed by Ofsted again and this time certified "Outstanding,"—the highest grade you could achieve! Nearly all my observations thereafter were certified "Outstanding" by Deputy Heads, Heads of Department, the Head teacher himself along with another Ofsted inspector with only a handful of "Goods" under my belt. The fact is, I was the bee's knees, and I knew it. I felt stable, comfortable, and loved my job more than anything else in the world.

Clearly, this concept of self-worth originated from the unremitting praise that extended over several years—my "looking-glass self."

One year into being a fully qualified teacher, I was promoted in my first school in Barnet, North London to Deputy Head of English. A while after that I was chosen to be placed onto the Outstanding Teacher Programme, which is a rare opportunity. This was an even greater ego boost for me as earning a place on this course certified me to coach other teachers to become "Outstanding". Don't even ask me what "Outstanding" means, I'm not sure anyone does, I'm not sure I ever did. I just knew despite my age and lack of life experience, I knew how to teach, how to bond with the students and how to plan and execute insightful lessons.

With my greater embedded confidence when the opportunity arose to finally be a Head of English, I jumped at the chance without any hesitation.

It was all I cared about. It was all I had shed blood, sweat and tears for.

I say I was naïve because I assumed with great responsibility came great power. How wrong I was. I was in charge of nine other amazing members of staff at this big but relatively new school in Enfield but worked twelve-to-thirteen-hour days, Monday through to Friday, taught Saturday school for the current Year 11s and faced masses of coursework to mark. This was all in addition to the day to day running of the department, ensuring I planned lessons efficiently and participating and sometimes leading endless meetings with staff, colleagues, deputy head, parents and dealing with students.

My head feels as if it is about to explode whilst re-telling this. I truly believed I would be able to make a difference, run the department in the best way possible, make my own decisions and attain full power to do what I thought was best for the students. How wrong I was.

I was respected by my department, I was respected by the students and hand on heart, the best part of the job was teaching them in the classroom. I guess I loved teaching because every day was different, every hour was different as I taught one class and then headed into another.

The students have remained embedded in my mind to this day; their voices echoing around the room as they actively participated and discussed the task. The looks of concentration conditioned in them as I observed their pens stroke the surfaces of their exercise books. The odd subservient look I would receive as they looked up at me in the silence, the reflective light from the projector resplendent on their faces.

If you ever want the truth about anything, teenagers are the best people to ask, they are rarely afraid to hurt your feelings and there is nothing subtle in voicing their opinions. So, hearing their regular feedback especially when it was positive and they enjoyed the lesson, only made me more in love with them than I already was. No one that goes into teaching hates children (and if they do, then they are definitely in the wrong job) so for me the children were the most enjoyable and rewarding part.

However, one day stress ravages you. It bites you, fills you with poison and gradually kills you. Kills your personality. Kills you as a person. Kills any interests you could or would want to have. Kills your spirit and enthusiasm and passion, until it grooms you along a dark path and you start to believe that nothing matters except your own problems.

The only memories that engulf you, are those of your own suffering.

It got to the stage whereby I became wholly consumed in work. The caretaker would often comment that my white Vauxhall Corsa was the first car in the car park and the last to leave. I was even warned by my Deputy Head in a meeting that I should avoid working so many hours, that they (senior management) 'wouldn't want me to burn out'.

I could not see any other way around it. I could not see another way out of it, it was the way I was conditioned to work. I lived every day in this manner, working every weekend and even when I wasn't working, thoughts of the week ahead consumed me. Yet, I refused to listen to anyone openly sharing their concerns. Yes, I was in a highly paid job, but I was starting to loathe it and unfortunately only I allowed the stress to take a toll on my mental and physical wellbeing. Only I had chosen this path.

What else could go wrong?

One day stress ravages you. It bites you, fills you with poison and gradually kills you.

*

The impact of the position and its responsibility were bad enough but, on top of everything, I fell in love with a colleague. A colleague who was married and had been with his wife for fifteen years.

No matter what you may think of me after reading this, sometimes you cannot help who you fall in love with. Sometimes you are in a relationship that isn't right and sometimes certain things are just not meant to be. But it doesn't make you a bad person. Sometimes morality is not black and white, and it is a situation you can only ever empathise with, if you've experienced it yourself.

At that time, it wasn't meant to be, and it certainly didn't help my mental state. He was confused but not able to leave his wife at the time. I became incredibly emotional, pining for our relationship to work. The lack of control I had, only added to feelings of entrapment. We were in an endless cycle. One moment we were the best of friends, lovers to the extent that we felt we could not be out of each other's sight. His classroom was only two doors down from mine and with the way I felt about him, it wasn't close enough.

L.

I wanted to be in his presence every second of the day, you could say I was borderline obsessed. Sometimes, I could sense his presence, whether he was about to pass my way, ambling down the corridor to use the photocopier outside my classroom, or sometimes I would receive a sensation in my gut and then I'd look up and he would be there, hovering in the doorway. His lean physique leant casually against the doorframe, eyes burning into mine, as he sometimes with an embarrassed countenance, fiddled nervously with his tie. His dress sense only made me idolise him more. We were so in tune with each other, we would predict the moment we would pass each other's way before it even happened.

Before I was to have my first lesson observation by the Deputy Head one cold, autumn morning, I walked nervously into my classroom and a hot coffee cup sat waiting for me on my desk. I touched the warm, smooth plastic and on the lid, in his handwriting, read: 'You are brilliant.' This was just one of many romantic gestures and it only solidified my deep love for him. I admired his boldness and his sensitivity. He was not the type of man who hid his feelings from me, and I loved that so much about him. I had never experienced this phenomenon with anyone else in my entire life, despite having been in love before. This was not the same. This felt so much deeper than lust and attraction. It was so many emotions combined into one; embarrassment, longing, nervousness, excitement, happiness. I almost felt we had met before, our passion, so familiar yet so unusual and something incredibly rare.

I was mesmerised; his face, his voice, his stance, his entire existence. During a non-teaching period, I would compulsively check the timetable system to see if he was teaching, just so I had an excuse to pass his way. I eventually knew his timetable off by heart. Once, I went as far to check his live running app (he ran most days) and haphazardly drove my car to a random country lane on a Saturday afternoon, just to speak to him even if just for five short minutes. The beaming smile on his face that day is stained in my memory.

Another memorable moment etched in my mind was an evening where we ended up strategically driving home at the same time. Both halted at a set of traffic lights during the twilight commute, me in my Corsa, him on his moped, he spontaneously and to my surprise got off his moped, lifted his helmet and leaned into my open window, holding my face in his hands and kissed me like he had never kissed me before. I never wanted the traffic signals to change. I wanted to be frozen in time. In that moment there ignited in me a rush of warmth and affection. The world around us was non-existent as we shared this brief but intimate connection. And as the lights changed to green, a curious onlooker in the car next to me looked with complete adoration and a huge smile on her face. I could read her mind; that she had never witnessed anything else so meaningful and romantic in her whole life, and just as I was, she was fully aware of how an action like this from him, spoke volumes of his love and the beauty of what we had, even in the most unexpected places.

He consumed every minute of my day. I was completely, utterly, unconditionally, in love with him.

In contrast, whilst in each other's company we would argue endlessly, sparked by our frustrations with the situation because we were so desperate to be together, but the odds were simply not in our favour. During this hideous cycle of our relationship, we would avoid speaking for days at a time (the longest I think was about four to six weeks) and then we would ride that same merry-go-round again. It made my head spin.

I had not one ounce of control over myself, my job, my emotional state and in fact my entire life. My whole day would be determined by the state *we* were in. It was on those days where we weren't speaking where my emotions would escalate, and I would feel my most vulnerable. My weakness would prevail, and, in those moments, I felt like Samson whose hair had been chopped off by the evil Delilah. Both my mental and physical strength had deteriorated and disappeared into an abyss. My stress would heighten, my concentration would diminish, and my only focus was on our unbearable situation. I only had tunnel vision for us. Looking back now, I realise how unhealthy this was.

My family suffer A LOT with their mental health. Whether that being depression, anxiety, OCD, agoraphobia, and many being on medication to get them through the day. It took my own father seventeen years to admit to me that he was suicidal when he and my mum divorced. His mental health deteriorated so much at the time, that my nan had to travel down to London from Newcastle and stay with him for three months to take care of him.

I never dreamed that I would develop any issues myself. I had never experienced anything like this before. If it wasn't for the few people closest to me at the time, I honestly do not know where I'd be now.

Would I even still be here?

To this day, biscuits remind me too much of this traumatic time; eating alone, being alone, living alone.

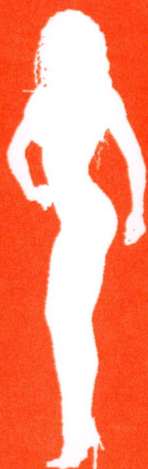

The pinnacle of my feelings occurred unexpectedly on my drive to work one day as I was talking to my best friend on the phone, which we were accustomed to doing every single day. Like a gunshot to my chest, my breathing became laboured, and I was panting uncontrollably. Failing to speak, my heart was racing; I was experiencing my first panic attack: (Mayo Clinic: "a sudden episode of intense fear that triggers severe physical reactions... you might think you're losing control." I wish I could tell you that this was the only time this occurred.

I sat in my car in the car park and felt so hysterical about starting the working day; I physically could not get out of the car.

To provide you with a better picture about how I was feeling, my relentless daily routine mirrored my unceasing emotional state. After a draining day at work, I would stop at the BP garage where I lived to purchase a ready meal (usually a Korma and a naan bread) and eat wearing just pyjamas, sometimes even in bed. I had no energy or motivation to even cook for myself, because I couldn't see any advantage to it. I was alone. Then, I'd go to sleep and watch something on my iPad. Despite having a whole two-bedroom rented house to myself, I'd only stay within the confines of my bedroom. I had become a recluse, a hermit.

My eating was all over the place; eating very little during the day and then binging in the evening. I recall on one occasion I scoffed two whole packets of biscuits and half a jar of Biscoff spread. Unsurprisingly, feeling bloated and then disgusted with myself, the guilt attacked me like a predator. These thoughts made a change from the negative ones about the job I had begun to hate. At the same time, I was grieving and mourning a relationship that was never going to be fully committed by L.

It made me feel so good, so comforted in the moment that I forgot all my woes as I relished the sweet sugar high. It was my temporary antidote. Digging deeper, all I was doing was harming myself by eating my emotions. To this day, biscuits remind me too much of this traumatic time; eating alone, being alone, living alone.

I knew my eating was becoming emotionally led because I would also binge at the weekends: "Researchers estimate that up to 60% of people who struggle with BED are women. The cause for the disorder is unknown, but there are likely social, biological and psychological factors." (Marcin, 2016) I sought solace and comfort in binging on snacks, sugary treats, cakes and takeaways; I didn't have the best relationship with food. It became something that I associated with relaxation, happiness and security. It made me feel elated in the moment and everyone knows when you eat your emotions, it can have a detrimental effect in the long run on your physical and mental wellbeing. These habits made me even more vulnerable and became a part of my newly adopted lifestyle.

In addition to these eating habits, my sleep was also starting to deteriorate and would often affect my mood, heightening my desire to overeat and binge: "Lack of sleep can create an imbalance in the body that increases ghrelin levels and lowers leptin levels. This can cause you to feel hungrier during the day." (Pacheco and Singh, 2023) There was no wonder I was hungry all the time! Stress combined with very bad sleep meant I was hungry ALL THE TIME.

At the peak of my stress, I would have repetitive sleep paralysis. For those of you who have never experienced this, it is the strangest experience, it almost feels paranormal. Sleep paralysis occurs when your sleep is very inconsistent, and your body has failed to recover effectively. What I'm about to relate is the closest I can to describe what it's like.

When you enter a deep sleep, your muscles completely relax and paralyse which is why you can sleep without acting out the actions in your dreams. What would happen to my body is that it would enter complete paralysis thinking it was asleep, but I was really awake. Some people hallucinate and I'm thankful I never experienced that. For me, I would try to move but I couldn't: "a temporary inability to move... a brief loss of muscle control known as atonia." (Suni, 2022)

The first time it happened was the scariest because it caused me great distress knowing there was nothing, I could do but to ride it out.

In addition to failing to move, there appeared a relentless humming, like a drone in my ear and every time it happened, it would feel as if my whole body was being raised to the ceiling. It was such a strange phenomenon I would believe my nose was touching it. I cannot even tell you how long it lasted. What felt like a few minutes, may have only been seconds. The frequency of these occurrences only diminished my fear and hence, my attitude became nonchalant, as it became a monthly expectation. The impending expectation dwindled its unsettling nature. I learnt to accept it until it passed.

Due to the frequency of these episodes, my mum was one of many people who became concerned about my health. Friends and other family members would inform me of their concerns, but I just ignored them and brushed it away. In the end, my mum persuaded me to see my GP so we could work out why it was happening so frequently.

When I eventually saw the GP, they wanted to refer me to a sleep specialist. Feelings of defeat rushed through me; my heart sank.

A week or so later I received the referral letter. As my eyes scanned the words on the page, I kept thinking that surely there must be a way that I could sort this out myself without having to go through a specialist. Whether denial, arrogance or laziness, when I received two letters reminding me to book in with the sleep specialist, I made the choice to ignore them both. I abandoned them, leaving them neglected and gathering dust on the shelf in the front porch.

As well as the sleep paralysis, I suffered with other sleepless nights filled with thinking and dreaming about work. Having two Year 11 classes and copious amounts of exam papers, homework and classwork to mark as well as their five pieces of coursework to complete, my anxiety was intensifying, and I was starting to feel suffocated by it: "High sleep reactivity is also linked to risk of shift-work disorder, depression and anxiety. Importantly, stress-related worry and rumination may exploit sensitive sleep systems… augmenting the pathogenicity of sleep reactivity." (Kalmbach, Anderson and Drake 2018)

Marking alone totalled 225 pieces of coursework. I also taught seven classes so being expected to mark their exercise books every three weeks was incredibly disheartening. Every set of books took three hours if done faultlessly. That's twenty-one hours of marking to complete within three weeks, on top of lesson planning which if done properly would take me about seven hours (I liked to plan for the whole week on a Saturday to relieve the stress and overall workload). Every task became impossible, and I was drowning. Sadly, many who remain in the teaching profession go through this turmoil every day.

How did I survive?

I felt the ultimate failure. Despite knowing I was a brilliant teacher, there were so many factors stopping me from staying one. Emphasis was no longer on the teaching or the students, it was all about hitting targets, securing numbers, attending pointless meetings, reading through at least fifty emails a day (no exaggeration when you're a Head of English!), dealing with student behaviour (rarely my own classes but other teachers in the department who were having issues), parent complaints, continuous scrutiny and observations…the list was endless. I no longer felt like the outstanding teacher I once was.

I was defeated.

Teaching had changed for the worse since I first trained in 2011. The focus at the start of my career was about embedding the love of learning in students, being creative with lessons and having freedom in the curriculum. Now, it was everything but.

Becoming a Head of English, as much as it felt like the greatest achievement of my life, proved to be my greatest downfall—my hubris. I knew six weeks into the job that I had to quit. I remember telling my best friend all the things I had discovered as soon as I got the job. It certainly wasn't the school that they made themselves out to be.

I discovered, all too late, my predecessor survived a mere six months, the woman before her three months and the time before that, the department didn't have anyone to fill the job for two academic years!

If you are a teacher reading this, I take my hat off to you. Maybe the guaranteed monthly pay check is why you keep calm and carry on, maybe the kids are the reason why you stay, even the naughty ones! No one ever pursues a career in teaching disliking children. They are the best part, and they are rarely the reason anyone chooses to leave, despite the common misconceptions about working with teenagers. They really made my day every day and if any of my former students are reading this now, thank you for brightening my days, my life and helping me carry on, even during my darkest times. It's crazy to think you have no idea how much of a positive impact you had on me. You truly kept me going year after year.

Regardless, teaching is such a thankless job. With more responsibility comes less power, more stress and when you try your hardest to work above and beyond, the goal posts change again, with demands and expectations on your time, energy and resources decreasing. Every year that passes causes you to feel that little bit more drained, that little bit more stressed, that little bit more anxious until you are bled dry and there is nothing more for you to give. You are a helpless, vulnerable, weak animal to the slaughter.

On top of the sleep paralysis and extremely high stress levels, my body started to react in other ways which looking back now, was due to this stress. For one, my periods started to become even more agonising every month; extremely heavy and with unbearable cramps: "Dysmenorrhea (i.e.: painful menstruation) people experiencing stress earlier in their cycle were more likely to report severe symptoms during the time leading up to and during menstruation." (Boutot, 2016)

On one occasion, I was hunched over my desk in the English office crying in pain. Colleagues were lovely and gave me a hot water bottle, realising I was unwell, yet worried so much what others would think of me if I dared request a leave of absence, so of course I never did. My anxiety proclaimed it laziness, not helped by the fact that everyone knew about the affair, and I believed my reputation was ruined.

Thoughts of how others viewed me, continued to taunt my mind; they would and could never understand how real the love was between L and I.

When you are at your most vulnerable, most weak and suffocated by your despair, the strength of human kindness causes you to realise how much good there is in the world.

When I wasn't on my cycle, I came to realise that my body was still trying to tell me that something was very wrong, yet I continued to ignore the signs. I started to bleed at random times of the month and the abominable cramps in my lower abdomen were not period pains. I recall during a non-teaching period having to walk down to reception desperate for some paracetamol and just ended up in the stock cupboard crying inconsolably from the pain, from the hurt, from everything.

To this day, I will never forget the kindness exhibited from Joy, one of the ladies who worked at reception. She undisputedly lived up to her name. She comforted me in the stock cupboard, held and hugged me and prayed for me. I was so overwhelmed with this kindness, reassured that people didn't hate or judge me, or view me as the scarlet woman or home wrecker. In that moment, she made me feel so comforted, I only wished I felt like this all the time. Joy was someone I didn't even know all that well, yet when you are at your most vulnerable, most weak and suffocated by your despair, the strength of human kindness causes you to realise how much good there is in the world.

So, what was I going to do about it?

After this, I knew I had to book a GP appointment for the unnecessary bleeding and was referred; three smear tests came back inconclusive, and I remember feeling so overwhelmed with anxiety.

I recall sitting in the waiting room that day, surrounded by women who had ovarian cancer and genuinely believing this was my fate. Waiting for what felt like a lifetime until my name was called, I glanced at one woman sitting in the corner, hands clasped together; dark, forlorn eyes, a lilac head scarf covering her bald head and sunken cheeks on her miniscule frame. Tears filled my eyes when the realisation came to me how precious life is and how it could just be taken away in a moment. Aspects of your life that consume you like work and relationships, mean nothing faced against death. Anton, my brother and best friend, waited patiently with me, holding my hand and reassuring me with kind words, proving to be the only person who in that moment truly stood by me, stable and consistent.

It was a loathsome experience. Having a camera pushed up your private parts, far from gentleness and sensitivity, was unnerving. The lovely nurses however attempted to calm me, advising me to stare at my anatomy on the screen, which added a bit of humour to the unpleasantness. But the pain persisted for the remainder of the appointment. Thankfully, it wasn't ovarian cancer; one of my walls had caved, causing the persistent bleeding. A deep sigh emitted from the pit of my stomach as the relief hit me. A massive weight had been lifted off my shoulders knowing it wasn't as serious as I believed it to be. Nevertheless, knowing what it *could have been* was enough to instil an everlasting fear within me.

A short while after that, I soon came to realise how amazing my department was and how much they liked and respected me. In my absence, they distributed my Year 11 exam papers, so I could recover and put myself first. I think that time was the first time I recognised that work could carry on without me. Lessons would still resume and the day to day running of the department and the school would still live to see another day.

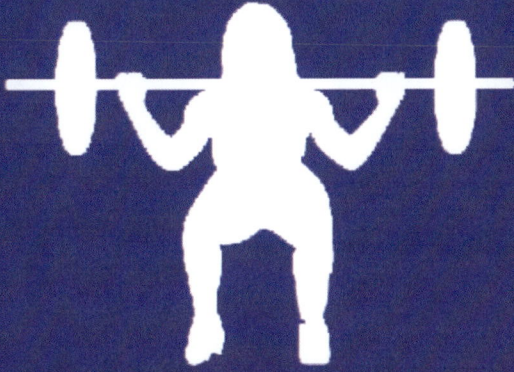

Aspects of your life that consume you like work and relationships, mean nothing faced against death.

Returning to work induced old habits. My illicit partner and I were still having our ups and downs; lovers and friends one minute, enemies and strangers the next. The last straw for me was in February (five months after we had met) when I discovered his purchase of a new house which he was to move into with his wife. He was moving in on a Friday (the next day) and I overheard him telling another colleague with excitement in the corridor, my ears drowning out everything but their conversation, my heart breaking.

The Instagram photo on my phone, an image of smiling excited faces surrounded by boxes and lovingly holding their dog, filled me with torment. It pained me to see his happiness. *I hated him. I hated her. I hated their happiness.* The distress and agony felt worse than my being murdered. This despair made me mourn him, for he had killed us, everything I had feared the most. It was this event that was the straw that broke the camel's back.

Due to my current mental state, I took a few sporadic days off work because I couldn't bear seeing him, on top of dealing with my own work. I just couldn't cope. Those days were a haze. I had no concept of time. I was a zombie merely breathing, but not fully functioning. Staying in bed all day, pyjama-clad, within the confines of my bedroom, only getting up to use the bathroom and to force something down me was the new routine. Instead, I found myself enveloped in a storm of frustration. Grabbing a pen and some paper, I began pouring my thoughts down, page after page after page. Each stroke of the pen was a release. As my feelings found refuge in the ink, the act of writing allowed me to dissect my emotions. Some pages serving as letters directly to him; a cathartic journey.

I had given up. On life, on me, on hope, on everything. I had come to the realisation and accepted that the relationship between us was never going to work, and this betrayal stung me, leaving me paralysed with the greatest grief, scarring me for a very long time.

I didn't know how to get myself out of this hellhole I was in and only I was to blame for getting myself into it. I was ensnared in this endless cycle of walking lethargically through my front door and crawling into bed, no matter how early it was until the next morning. It would be odd if I had a day where I didn't cry. Other than speaking to my mum who would ring me daily and my best friend, I became flaky as a person; a person I didn't recognise. I would make arrangements with others only to cancel at the last minute because I just wasn't up to it physically or mentally. The motivation to interact with others was simply non-existent. I probably only kept in contact with a few people I could count on one hand and as I gradually became more detached, my circle became smaller and smaller. I would indulge in big portions of food because it emanated my only comfort. I was on a carousel of being in high spirits when I overindulged, yet undereating and dropping weight when distraught. There was no structure or stability to my life in any form.

I'm so ashamed to admit this, but when emotions were at their lowest, I would often take Night Nurse or travel sickness tablets before bed because it meant if I was knocked out, I would get a decent night's sleep; I was subsequently numb to any negative emotions. I could not cry; I could not feel.

This I have NEVER revealed, but suicidal thoughts ran through my head during this time. Although I knew deep down, I would *never* put any action to these thoughts, they still entered my mind, simply because I was at the bottom of the pit of despair and desperate to escape, not knowing which way to go or how to climb out. There were moments where I wished I was brave enough to act on them.

My mental health was declining with every passing day because of the job and the fact he and I were not on good terms.

Two days are stained in my memory.

Like a volcano, out of nowhere, I erupted. I was so angry with him for not choosing me that I attempted to burn all his letters, cards and gifts in the log burner, situated on the fading patio in the back garden. A few of the paper notes ignited but I remember screaming out of frustration on the phone to my best friend, not caring what my neighbours thought as I watched in anticipation, the *Wuthering Heights* novel he had gifted me, go up in flames. To my surprise, it failed to burn. Hands shaking, my heart bursting out of my chest with panic, I kept trying to light it, my thumb shakily flicking the lighter again! And again! And again! Yet to no avail.

I was someone I did not recognise and felt like a mental woman, a bunny boiler you see in those B movies on Netflix, completely out of control. I looked as if an evil spirit possessed me. When I think back now, I feel embarrassed, ashamed and shocked that this relationship and the job I hated had turned me into this. A monster. This was not me; I did not recognise myself. My best friend was so worried she said she was scared I would burn the house down and pleaded to come over, but I persuaded her not to. Eventually I calmed down and returned to my bedroom, hiding away distressed yet silent, like a vulnerable animal crawling back into their hideaway.

The other most significant day was a day where yet again, I couldn't face going into work. Anton came round knowing the state I was in. I hadn't left the bedroom, and I didn't even have the mental or physical energy to open the front door for him on his arrival, he simply let himself in with his key.

This was the day of the Magic Moment, and I will never forget it.

With exhaustion and despair, Anton sat at the end of my bed, relentlessly pronouncing his concerns that I could not carry on like this. I wasn't living any sort of life. Instead, he posed the question: 'Tash, why don't you start weight training with me? It will give you something to do after work, like a hobby and it will clear your head.'

I sunk into my duvet thinking weight training, how is that going to solve anything? How would it ever change my situation or my feelings?

I told him I would have to think about it and although it sounded like an excuse, I explained that I needed to feel ready before I committed.

The truth is those golden words remained in my head. Although Anton never mentioned it again, quite a few months went by and after contemplating it enough, out of the blue one day I said I would give it a try. Little did I know that this decision was to absolutely transform my life. *Forever.*

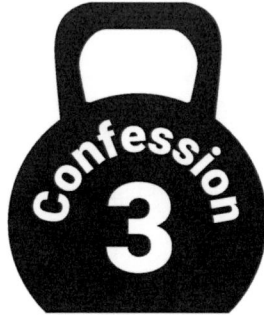

What Training Was

"When you go through hardships and decide not to surrender, that is strength."
Arnold Schwarzenegger

You never forget the feelings of accomplishment when you swim without armbands. You never forget your first day at secondary school; uniform neat and pressed, shiny black shoes so pristine your face reflects radiantly from the crown; that fear in the pit of your stomach rupturing the closer you saunter to the gates. You never forget the day you pass your driving test and embrace that torrent of freedom, feeling like you could walk on air because you now retain full independence and liberation. You never forget your first love.

My first weight training session with Anton was no different to these other milestones in life, that transform you indefinitely and I remember this rite of passage as clear as day.

I reminisce walking through the doors of the gym studio irresolutely, feeling anxious, nervous, dubious of what to expect or how to even feel, out of my depth. In awe of my surroundings, I observed men exerting themselves, their sweaty chins caressing the bars as they executed pullups, women in full rigour squatting an unthinkable amount of weight, the booming sound of the playlist resonating through my ears and discerning this look on everyone's faces; a look of fatigue, accomplishment and focus. Every individual was captured in their zone. For the first time in a long time, I was a complete beginner. Putting myself in an environment like this one where I felt inferior and uncomfortable was something I was not used to, and I didn't quite know how to feel about it.

I can't say I enjoyed my first session as such. I remember attempting a barbell squat for the first time and Anton having to put a foam roller and pad down because my depth was appalling and I needed something to aim for, as he attempted to teach me the technique for the first time. To this day, I fail to recall other exercises we completed, it all feels such a blur, but what I will never forget was the excruciating pain reverberating my whole body the next day, the day after and the day after that, also known as DOMS (Delayed Onset Muscle Soreness). "Delayed-onset muscle soreness (DOMS) is usually observed 12-24 hours following unaccustomed strenuous exercise...The soreness increases to a peak between 24 and 72 hours then subsides by 7 days." (Lee and Healy 2011) In fact, the pain of tenderness in my joints, soreness in my muscles and agony of my entire being lasted a whole week!

My whole body felt in complete and utter pain, so bad I almost felt numb to it.

I was supposed to have another session that week and I informed Anton that I wished to cancel because I could barely walk. It was the most unendurable pain I've ever felt. Getting out of bed, something I took for granted everyday was strenuous. My legs felt like a bag of bricks, like permanent shackles around my ankles and any physical day to day task was oppressive. Funnily enough, Anton confirmed we wouldn't cancel, he would just adapt that second session to upper body exercises. There was no getting out of that one, authenticating his role as the ultimate task master.

The more I trained, the more I revelled in it as I saw progression when my weights increased every week. The pain in the sessions was so much more bearable than the pain and stress from work and everything else going on in my head. I took myself by surprise and after a period I was anticipating our next session. It was a different kind of accomplishment, knowing I was advancing in something I knew nothing about, completely blind to where this yellow brick road was leading me. All I knew was how it made me feel in the moment. I loved that feeling it gave me.

The pain in the sessions was so much more bearable than the pain and stress from work and everything else going on in my head.

Enjoyment flourished.

I requested increasing my sessions to four times a week. Anton was so pleased at my suggestion and explained I would now have a proper split with two lower body days and two upper body days; muscle specific training sessions. This was how it stayed for a couple of years. Training was carefully executed and meticulously planned, and I was learning more and more as the months went on. My strength was hitting the roof, week after week, month after month and soon I started to become recognised as "Anton's sister" the "strong sister".

Despite becoming more confident with the exercises, I was still wearing very unattractive gym gear (baggy washed out tracksuit bottoms and hideous t-shirts) because I didn't own a pair of leggings, nor did I have the body confidence or esteem to portray myself otherwise. Fundamentally, I wasn't yet "good enough" to be like everyone else or look like every other attractive woman on the gym floor. I laugh now when I remember Anton saying jokingly, 'Well, you need to start wearing better gym clothes now', simply because I didn't own any and my clothing did not reflect my capabilities. Self-assurance grew like vines within me and as I started to dress more confidently, I was being recognised and noticed. Self-worth transpired for the first time in a long time since becoming an "outstanding" teacher.

For once, others were looking in awe at *me*. The progression from a trap bar deadlift (lifting a heavy weight from the floor using a big, metal rack, important for beginners) to a barbell one (the progression lift using a 20kg metal pole) was a huge momentous breakthrough. The first time I hit 80kg on a sumo deadlift (again, using a barbell) I had an audience who all stopped in their tracks to observe the execution. I recall an explosion of applause as I finished, and it made me feel so good. For the first time in a long time, I felt genuinely happy.

My barbell squats (squatting placing the barbell on your back) were improving and I no longer needed a target like a bench to hit depth and was starting to squat 70kg with ease, then eventually 80kg. As my upper body strength started to ameliorate, my banded dips (lifting your whole bodyweight in a push up position off two bars) eventually moved onto bodyweight and one of the biggest achievements for me was hitting my first bodyweight pullup (pulling yourself up by holding bars).

I still possess many videos that tell the story of my fitness journey and quite a few on my pullup journey. In one, I am in a white band (the thinnest one) to which Anton announces, 'soon you won't be using a band'. I still surprise myself now with how far I've come, thinking about what were once the biggest hurdles are now second nature to me. Of course, my first bodyweight pullups exhibited terrible form, but it is crazy to think I managed it in the end; it took two whole years of consistent training to achieve it. Some people never do.

Another funny video I have is me pushing Anton on the prowler (a heavy piece of exercise equipment which you push in laps), that certainly got a few laughs. At the time he weighed about 80kg, not to mention the added 20kg plates that were on it! I thought he was joking when he said that was my finisher, but God did I do it. In fact, there was nothing I didn't do. I didn't complain and I faced every challenge, every new exercise. I wanted to try *everything* to get better, to prove I was good enough, to myself but also to win Anton's approval. The feeling was indescribable.

As I continued to get noticed by clients and trainers alike, I couldn't help embracing the incessant compliments. I was lifting heavier than most clients and even the female PTs there! For the first time, I no longer felt inferior, nor out of place or uncomfortable. Thriving on the hope that this was my last chance to heal myself, it only drove my motivation.

I am bewildered with how different my attitude was on the day of the "magic moment". I no longer felt the need to hibernate in my bedroom, I now had a purpose. It was as if someone had injected me with complete euphoria. My growing positivity was not linear, but overall, it was growing within me the more time wore on.

My nutrition still had to be augmented, a vital aspect of fitness I messed up on many occasions. Once, I stupidly trained the day after I binged greedily on chocolate, a habit I struggled to remove myself from. I felt so awful the next day in the session; weaker, fatigued and my performance was terrible, inducing another feeling of failure.

On another occasion, I made the mistake of having too much protein beforehand and my stomach felt so bloated, like a balloon that could be popped any second, with any given movement. Every exercise felt difficult.

Though incredibly rare, I remember having a drinking session the night before and trained with a bad hangover. Little did I know at the time that Anton pushed me even harder and showed zero sympathy towards such foolishness. The sickness rose instantaneously after every set. I was learning more and more about myself and the choices I was making. The two certainly didn't go hand in hand. It was only from learning from these mistakes that the penny dropped, and realisation kicked in that if performance and training were that important to me, then I would have to change my nutrition and habits once and for all. Poor eating was determining bad sessions and feeling fatigue and sluggish was not going to impress Anton, so I knew I needed to change.

Eventually I made that step to focus on my nutrition. A wealth of knowledge enthralled me. I came to learn and understand calories and macronutrients (carbohydrates, fats, and proteins). I endured trials and errors with snacks so I could figure out what would optimise my performance. Sometimes a banana was too little if I hadn't eaten since lunchtime and I was training at 6 p.m. Protein cookies were too protein heavy, shakes were not carb heavy enough. I think I went through a stage of having sweets (even though I hated them) beforehand and then eventually devouring five marshmallows directly before a session. But I got there in the end. Eventually I started having a mini meal beforehand like a bowl of oats with a banana and a shake and I started to notice that I was properly fuelled for the session ahead. Advanced preparation married with routine became my new lifestyle.

As the care for my nutrition and body began to improve, so did my sleep. The sleep paralysis soon disappeared. My mood improved. My down days lessened and although I still had them occasionally, I learnt to deal with them better. With an improved mood came an improved confidence and a more positive attitude.

During a rest period in one of my sessions, Anton recalled, 'Tash, do you remember before you started training and you said you wanted to, but you had to be "ready?" I knew you would'. I don't think I even replied, I merely allowed his kind words to sink in. I may have said 'I know,' quietly under my breath, my smile not leaving my face, embracing this new person I had become. I couldn't believe at that moment how far I had come, not just in my performance, but in how I felt; a totally different person mentally. I was reborn.

The day where I got tricked into a Personal Best (a weight you've never lifted before) was a day of complete exultance. We were using the main deadlift platform in the studio, so it was one of those days where *I knew I could not fail*. The platform was positioned in the centre of the gym, so all eyes were on me. Every individual from every corner of the room would be able to see. It fell to either one of two things. Either Anton was clumsy in miscalculating the number of plates he had put on, or he had done it deliberately in a calculating way to push me to succeed. To this day, I still have no idea.

But it led to this pivotal moment.

I would rarely ask how much was on the bar because at times my nerves got the better of me. Focusing on the lift itself and getting through it was all I could do. At this point, I thought I was lifting 110kg. Unbeknownst to me, it was in fact a whopping 120kg and he was recording this focal moment on his phone. On this day, I came to realise the strength of my mind.

I stepped uneasily onto the jet-black platform. My hands clutched at the ice-cold treasure of a barbell. I placed my wraps around my wrists like a suit of armour before heading into battle and braced myself for the initial lift as my adrenaline pumped a hundred miles an hour through my entire body. My stomach was performing a mountain of somersaults and as the beautiful sound of the bar rang through my ears, it expertly kissed the platform with every rep and on finishing, I felt complete relief and gratification. Afterwards, I was speechless; failed to even comment on how heavy it was, which showed how confident I felt.

Anton knew what it would have done to me if he had revealed it was a Personal Best. On a few occasions prior to hitting PBs, I would feel sick rise to my throat before a deadlift and other times my hands would be shaking so much, I would struggle to grip the bar. I don't think he could ever understand why I was so nervous, nor did I. It was just the way my body reacted. How clever the human mind is. My thinking I had lifted the weight before, had diminished any fear and self-doubt I may have otherwise had. I had succeeded!

Training became embedded in me. It was something I did without fail four times a week and became something I couldn't live without. It was a part of me, my identity. Not only did I become stronger in the gym, I started to become stronger as a person. I stopped worrying about things so much at work and started to accept there was nothing I could do about other people, or decisions made that were out of my control. You could say I started caring less because training was at the top of my priority list now. Whether this was good or bad I don't know, but it meant I wasn't as anxious and I was seeing the benefits to my mental and physical health over not being at work. Although on occasion I still got incredibly stressed, it was never as bad as the day of the panic attack.

Training became embedded in me. It was something I did without fail four times a week and became something I couldn't live without. It was a part of me, my identity.

Training helped me survive when other bad things happened, but like I said, I was coping better with training, than without. By feeling more confident and stronger as a person through training, I was finally realising my worth.

I concluded that being a Head of English was not for me, nor feasible for me to carry on living life in this way. So, without another job to go to, I apprehensively handed in my notice a few days before the deadline; I'd only survived a mere 8 months in this role. Despite my head teacher's attempts to persuade me to stay, I stood my ground; my decision was final.

Admittedly, my pride was hurt; I had failed at something that I had worked so arduously for. Word had travelled around, and I was faced with probing questions daily from other members of staff such as, 'Wow, where are you going next?' to which I would reply 'I don't have a job yet'. People's immediate reactions were of shock and on numerous occasions was told I was "brave."

I was brave.

By feeling more confident and stronger as a person through training, I was finally realising my worth.

Those were the
most painful five
months of my life.

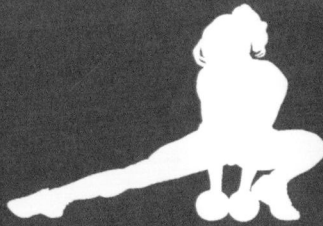

The emptiness I felt
left me permanently
hollow. I was altered
as a person, numb
and cold.

No one did that. No one gave up a highly paid salary as a Head of English with nothing to go to and still have rent to pay, a car to pay for, bills to pay. Not to mention, I was single and living alone and there was no one I could rely on financially. In my head, I felt anything was better than staying. What was even more telling was the fact that at the same time I left, another two people in my department did too. You could call it a domino effect. This often happens in the teaching world.

I informed L I was leaving, which only heightened the emptiness and heartbreak that came with it. By this point he had recently separated from his wife after she discovered our 'relationship' and it was very unclear where it left us. Things were too raw. We tried to make a go of it, but it didn't last. Shortly after I left the school, we agreed to separate permanently with no contact thereafter.

Those were the most painful five months of my life.

The emptiness I felt left me permanently hollow. I was altered as a person, numb and cold. Training really did save me during this time and remained the only stable element of my life and so I gripped it tightly with everything I had in me. Of course, I was still incredibly low, crying every day, feeling lonely but training helped me cope; my lifeboat, my last thread. It was the only consistent thing in my life. It helped me escape the deepest heartbreak I have ever felt. Trust me when I say, I cried more over L than I have done in any other relationship I had ever had previously. I don't know what it was about him. But having training to focus on, helped me, or rather *forced me* to learn to live without him, my last attempt at survival.

One cold, winter morning in January 2017, I walked out to find my car encased in a thick layer of frost. Armed with a scraper, I worked methodically to clear the ice, feeling the chill seep into my gloves despite the urgency to get going and avoid being late for work. Yet, I froze in surprise. There, etched on the bonnet was a love heart with our initials delicately intertwined. Seeing this unexpected gesture by him was a poignant reminder of the affection we once shared, prompting me to reflect on the significance of what this action meant.

What was his expectation, a reaction? An attempt for me to contact him? Despite his action of a reminder of a love we once had, I knew I couldn't open that door again. The past had to remain where it was, even as his love still lingered on the front of my car. I knew what I had to do.

Absolutely nothing.

One month later, the 11th February 2017.

My life was one of routine and military precision. I was either at the gym, at work or at home. This day changed everything, my whole future. In those last five months I tried to get on with my life, to stay afloat amongst the hardships of a failed relationship and a job I loathed. I had a new job in Essex that I had started five months previously and I hadn't heard from L in all that time. I never had the heart to delete or block his number, but I had no ties to him either. I had no idea where he was, how he was, the position he was in, if he was well or anything else. Unscrupulously, these thoughts would enter my head, but I would avoid overthinking for fear of setting me off emotionally.

The day we had parted was the end for me as far as I was concerned. Yet, to my surprise as I walked out of the gym studio that day feeling invigorated from the endorphins and a spring in my step, my phone told me I had two missed calls from him, his name and matching picture flashing on the face of my home screen.

I nearly dropped my phone. I was so shocked; my hands shaking.

An explosion detonated in my head. I was shell shocked. Strangely enough, I didn't react in the way I used to previously whereby a mountain of tears would ensue and without hesitation would have rushed to phone him back. The truth was, in addition to my shock, I felt a sense of anger.

How dare he disrupt a life I had started to fix?

How dare he attempt to ruin the stability I had slogged so hard to achieve?

I had just got my life on track, I was finally starting to move on and accept that things never worked between us, but I questioned whether it was right to return his call. I didn't want to revert to my former, weaker self when I was around him, I did not like "me" back then, feeling like I *needed* him, allowing him that amount of power over me.

Training was my one true love, it was the one thing that could never hurt me (well not permanently), and I liked who I was now; someone happier, comfortably independent, confident and embracing my new life routines.

My body sunk deeply into the seat of my car. Despair, defeat, and uncertainty casting a spell in my mind. I sat frozen staring at my phone, seriously contemplating whether I should call him back. It could have been five minutes or twenty, time had stood still while I struggled to decide. Subconsciously, my thumb pressed the green button, and those rings caused a pang of sickness to rise in my throat.

Although I was altered, his voice brought back great joy and a feeling of elation when he answered. There were many silences and rasped pauses in this short conversation, yet it was more of a casual conversation between two friends that were catching up, not of two people still hopelessly in love who hadn't seen each other in five months. Although L suggested meeting, a part of me didn't want to go back there. I was cautious and hesitant. I felt I was a better person now, a stronger one, he only made me weak and reminded me of the most painful time in my life. I agreed to meet but was on my guard.

The day I saw him again for the first time, felt completely surreal.

Training was my one true love, it was the one thing that could never hurt me.

I was early, sitting and waiting in the local Costa, ringing my sweaty palms together underneath the table.

My head unremittingly glanced up every time I heard the door swing open, my heart sinking that it wasn't him. The cold, February breeze caused goosebumps on my arms and on my exposed ankles and I was so nervous. As another breeze entered the shop, a glimpse of a man caught my eye and my eyes shot up. I gazed, completely mesmerised.

I saw him.

He waded in, his patterned scarf swaying behind his left shoulder as the wind blustered and a beaming smile emanated from him as our eyes locked.

It was as if no time had passed at all. In that moment of greeting, we had reverted to *us* of five months previous. Echoes of strangers' voices and the clatter of cups on saucers faded, and he and I were the only two beings in that whole place. That day he made a promise, which he managed to keep for the remaining years we had together: "One day I will break down this brick wall around you, no matter how long it takes."

He knew I was altered. He knew I was no longer weak; he knew I had self-worth, and he knew he had to prove himself *to me*.

Training was and still is everything to me. No matter what happened back then and no matter what life throws at me now. Like water, it keeps me living, like air it keeps me breathing. It made me so much stronger as a person that it took L a long time to work his way back into my life, he had to earn that right.

The "brick wall" which he described on many occasions at the time, took many months to knock down, yet he kept reassuring me he would eventually succeed, brick by brick. I slowly started to open my heart to him again.

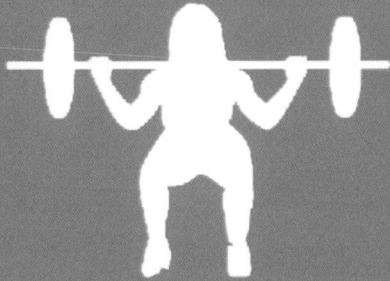

Training was and still is everything to me. No matter what happened back then and no matter what life throws at me now. Like water, it keeps me living, like air it keeps me breathing.

I had the upper hand for the first time, I held all the cards. Everything was on my terms now. No one *ever again* was going to make me unhappy or treat me in a way I didn't deserve and if they did, they would be quickly annihilated.

Training transformed my personality. It made me who I am now and embedded in me the self-worth I was lacking for so many years. It healed and cured me.

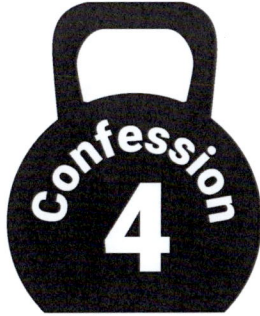

Inspirations

"Each person must live their life as a role model for others."
Rosa Parks

The consistency of training over a long period of time, embedded itself into my entire being and very quickly became my identity. My complete existence started to veer closer towards this idea of competing, but the seed was not planted straight away. There are always catalysts to your future actions; a moment, a person, an epiphany, a decision, all pushing you towards a life changing action.

I think it fair to say that Anton was probably my biggest inspiration. He still is. He *was* the training; he *was* the discipline; he *was* the enthusiast; the passion maker; the success. He embedded a confidence in me, he instilled this idea that my progression in the gym was limitless, and he didn't even know he was consciously doing it, that's what made him so endearing.

There are always catalysts to your future actions; a moment, a person, an epiphany, a decision, all pushing you towards a life changing action.

The passion I would see in his eyes when he trained his clients and even when he trained me, was phenomenal. I sensed his elation in the moments of my observation, the focus and the drive within him, mirroring his client. Watching him compete in 2017 only epitomised this fact. I watched in awe from the stand as he glided across the stage, the music booming through my eardrums, orchestrating the cheers from every single person in the arena. In that exact moment, he had made it.

Screaming at the top of my lungs, I rose from my chair in applause. I was injected with adrenaline, and tears of joy stung my eyes. He became a Pro straight away, placing 3rd and 2nd in his category; withstanding an absence of doubt that he would be successful hereafter.

Walking nervously into the arena that day, unsure of what to expect, feelings of discomposure swept over me, pondering how strange it all was. Encircling me were muscly, orange-tanned individuals in glittering bikinis and tight pants, bright reflections of diamonds and the smell of sweat, combined with the heat of bodies and damp skin.

Observing these surroundings only made me feel more of an outsider. Yet, we were the voyeurs of these other beings. I didn't belong, I didn't seem normal either compared to them. Glancing at the women who looked like they had just strut down a catwalk, infused me with aspiration. I knew at that moment I wanted to achieve something like this, a once in a lifetime experience which only a handful of people could ever have. Little did I know that in just over two years that would be me, *us*-me and Anton competing together at this exact arena, on this exact day.

The thing is, I thought I understood how difficult the process was for Anton to compete, but really, I couldn't have been any further from understanding and I now laugh sarcastically to myself at my naivety. All I knew was Anton was on a specific diet, which meant he couldn't eat the same meals as us at dinner or eat out at restaurants and that's all I thought it entailed. What I was to come to realise two years later, were all the hidden secrets around competing in bodybuilding, the mental and emotional turmoil you endure both during and after.

The first time this awareness arose was an episode I witnessed; one of his many post-show binges: "Extended periods of restrictive dieting is a common practice amongst bodybuilders preparing for a competition. We have found that post competition, bodybuilders fall into a trap of binge eating which leads to weight gain and depression." (Davidson, et al., 2017)

At the time it was something we all laughed at, but looking back now, he was in a very dark place, and it should never have been taken lightly, or chortled at.

We were at our mum's house a few weeks after his last show in 2017 and after a delicious dinner, we were all gathered in the living room for our evening dessert. As my eyes veered from the TV to my mum's face we continued to engage in conversation. I couldn't help but notice Anton leaving the room numerous times to go to the kitchen. I stepped inquisitively into the kitchen and to my surprise, discovered him frantically raiding my mum's cupboards, but at the same time, I didn't pay much attention to his hankering as he searched the cupboards with urgency.

None of us were aware how much he was consuming, but within ten or so minutes of engaging in conversation with him, he stopped. His face looked near enough to pass out. He slid down sitting sluggishly on the cold, beige tiled floor in a food coma, looking and feeling sick. His head was leant back against one of the bottom cupboards, his eyes weary as if he had been drugged. My response was to laugh, but knowing what I know now, experiencing what I've experienced, I would never have reacted in such a way if I could go back. It fills me with pain and guilt, knowing I have lived that exact moment too many times and yet in that second, saw the humour rather than the seriousness of it.

I was helpless in the moment and didn't know how to respond to his seemingly unusual behaviour. He went through what every bodybuilder post show goes through; uncontrollable and relentless binges and more, the physical changes not even near as painful as the mental devastation and trauma that stays with you. Yet, these behaviours are and remain a taboo, kept secret and never spoken about publicly in the world of competing. Suffering in silence is your only avenue and diction.

At the end of 2018, Anton had an article published in *Muscle and Fitness Magazine,* an edition with Arnold Schwarzenegger on the front cover, and one of the biggest names in the bodybuilding world. My brother was already on the highest pedestal imaginable, my feelings of pride unlimited. I bought three copies from WH Smith in King's Cross where I was meeting friends for the day and couldn't help boasting to them of his success.

I wanted to be just like him. I wanted *his* life. The irony was, I was the teacher with the 2:1 degree in English and he had published a written piece before me! Of course, he had allowed me to help him through the editing stages, so I can take some of the credit at least. But him being interviewed on podcasts, being a part of the Grenade team (the biggest and most successful protein bar company in the world), just monumented his success. Even today in everything he does, he is that individual that always strives to be better, his personal growth endless in its transformation. How he has grown and embraced fulfilment and enjoyment in everything he does, is something I will always admire; traits many desire but rarely ever attain.

Another inspiration of mine was a female powerlifter who worked briefly at the gym studio I was working at. Her strength was unbelievable, I don't think I have ever seen any other female lift like her, she was a real-life superwoman. She was one of the girlfriends at the time of another PT and I remember browsing her Instagram page in astonishment for hours, even showing my friends how much I wanted to be her. She was deadlifting a crazy amount of weight (I think over 160kg), benching probably 100kg if not more and I was in complete and utter awe of her.

In a conversation with Anton one evening, I exposed my excitement and admiration of her. I craved her strength, her look, her confidence and assuredly expressed my goal of being a powerlifter just like her. My only delight was Anton's reassurance of his belief that my strength was beyond that of the average female. This idea of powerlifting seemed appealing, as it didn't involve aesthetics or getting to an unnatural leanness, so no judgement of appearance in this sport was apparent.

I was so driven to be strong exactly like her, I would ponder it during most training sessions, wanting to push myself further, especially when I observed her training in the corner of the studio. Her hair gracefully whipping across her face with every rep she took, making it look so easy. Even her beads of sweat looked elegant and her whole body was smooth and in sync with the movement. Her level of control caused me to stop in reverence. My astonishment at how immeasurable female strength could be, only drove me deeper into the weightlifting game.

As my knowledge of nutrition improved, I started my first mini cut (a calorie- controlled diet to drop bodyfat) around 2017 which I believe lasted maybe ten or so weeks and I got down to my lowest weight at that time of 129lbs. People started to notice the transformation in my physique, and it only drove my motivation and kept me in high spirits. By doing this, it was the first time I had built an education around macros and calories. Once I understood how to track and weigh my food, it became much easier to stick to. I was really starting to be noticed at this point and I was relishing the attention.

Anton would start putting our training sessions on his Instastories and he would share with me the many replies of admiration. I just could not believe that this time, people were looking *at me* in awe, not the other way round, and not just for my strength but my physique.

It was such a self-esteem booster. Yet, there would still be the little voice in my head questioning whether I deserved people to notice me. I wasn't special or talented, yet to others I was important enough to be noticed and, in some ways, the less confident Tash still viewed myself as something less than average.

Despite the change my body was going through, that little voice lingered, that insufferable bad mindset, telling me I could never be good enough. It was as if there were two of me, fighting and battling it out.

Other clients training at the same time would utter comments like: 'Wow, you look lean', to which Anton would respond with good humour, 'Yeah, she looks like she trains now.' It was only until two of the best PTs in the studio made a comment that planted the seed in my head, which never disappeared. Neither of these male PTs said it to me personally, but one (the owner), mentioned to Anton assuredly, 'Your sister could do a show'. The only phrase I did get from him in person was, 'Wow you've never been this weight,' which was his idea of a compliment, and this guy *never* gave out compliments. With a beaming smile on my face, I replied 'No, never,' whilst at the same time his client agreed and commented on my leanness.

This was another turning point in my fitness career, and I had achieved a lean, toned physique for the first time. Another PT went on to tell Anton, 'Your sister could compete' and I think once in the gym he asked if I was, and I laughed it off in embarrassment.

It got to the stage where because my body had transformed so much, many clients would assume this was the case. My immediate reaction was always to exclaim how much the thought humoured me and I would dismiss it with the statement, 'No, I'm not good enough,' to which the conversation would be shut down immediately.

It was as if there were two of me, fighting and battling it out.

Although I had built up a lot of confidence, there was still a huge part of me that kept thinking I would never be good enough to do it. But everyone knows when enough people say the same thing, it makes you question and realise they are telling the truth and it becomes manifested in your brain. I was curious whether it would ever be something I could accomplish, even if it appeared unachievable.

It was a night out with two of my girlfriends in London's King's Cross (Camino's to be exact) where I had already made my decision that this was what I was destined to do. They asked with excited faces: 'Are you going to do it?! Are you going to compete?!' Abruptly I said, 'No, way, I've told you, I'm not good enough, why do people keep asking me?!' with a slight hint of annoyance. One of them told me not to be ridiculous and in a way, you could say that she was the one that made my decision for me, or rather bullied me closer towards it. Without hesitation, she messaged my brother there and then, whilst we were sat casually by the bar, sipping our cocktails. Feeling the tingle of the Sangria on my lips, she flashed her phone in front of my face as I observed the message: *'Your sister is going to compete'*. I simply laughed it off, my own brother, the person I was closest to in this whole world, did not know how much I really wanted to walk this path. She even went as far as going on the website, repeatedly flaunting her phone excitedly in front of my face. Seeing those women in bikinis, looking tanned and in amazing condition, made my heart soar.

I can't remember how long after, but in one of my sessions, I worked up the courage to tell Anton my ambition. He smiled, gave a little laugh and said he didn't want me to. The moment turned from electrifying and uncontrollable excitement to a blunt, flat, gut-wrenching, cold atmosphere. I was gutted. I was unsure whether it meant I wasn't good enough, or whether he thought I would simply try and then fail.

He explained that what it involved was so much more than just dropping the weight; only now do I know why this was his initial reaction. He was so honest and informed me of where the difficulty really lay, the aftermath. He explained I would never look at food in the same way again, food would become numbers, not to mention the impact it would have on my health, my periods: "Tash, everything about food will just become numbers to you, you won't look at things in the same way, *ever again.*" Ironically, as a coach now, whenever anyone enquires about the prospect of me coaching them for shows, I subtly dissuade them, echoing the same protective wisdom my brother once shared with me. However, if those individuals remain undeterred, I recognise their unwavering dedication and passion are genuine and they are truly ready for the level of commitment required.

His words only drove my hunger for it and the rebel within me was pushing. Anton resolved that I would have to put two years aside as I didn't have nearly enough muscle to be good enough to step on stage. He said I would have to complete a muscle building phase, which would involve me putting on weight and whether that would be a problem for me. I remember my exact words in affirmation: 'I know you don't want me to do it, but I don't care how long it takes me, it's all I want.' In defeat, he smiled and asserted, 'OK, fine, we start a building phase Monday.' I was so excited to begin this journey and I knew I had the best coach behind me.

I enjoyed the building phase so much. It was only towards the end where the enjoyment started to taper out, I became sick of food. What was once a pleasure, became a gradual resentment. It was a real struggle chewing meals and swallowing when I wasn't hungry: "During the off-season, it is advantageous for the bodybuilder to be in positive energy balance so that extra energy is available for muscle anabolism... adequate protein must be available to provide amino acids for protein synthesis." (Lambert, 2004) It was at its closure that I was embracing this idea of a long-term diet. I felt sluggish and fat and I wanted to feel good again. Every meal that became more difficult, only drove my motivation to ascertain the Holy Grail. Every unwanted bite reminded me of how much muscle I craved and how I wanted to look the best I could be on stage.

His words only drove my hunger for it and the rebel within me was pushing.

My strength and performance for the most part was at its peak. There were various challenges in the studio for clients and I remember beating all the women in the prowler push challenge (78m).

I was becoming so confident at training, Anton turned around to me one day and said, 'Tash, you don't need me anymore, you can train yourself now.' Shock and upset pervaded and in desperation I replied, 'No, no, I need you!' To which he said with reassurance, 'No you don't.'

I think it was at this point that I dropped my sessions with Anton from four to two. The plan was I would do all the difficult exercises with him, such as barbell squats and deadlifts, and I would do the more bearable exercises in my own sessions, using dumbbells for accessories and even machines, which were easy enough to do independently.

The very first session I completed solo is one I will never forget. I was literally shaking with fear and my stomach was doing a mountain of somersaults because I felt so intimidated about going into the weights section of the gym by myself. No one to spot me, no one to coach me on the movements, no one to guide me if I was doing anything wrong, or if my hand or foot were in the wrong position. I was alone, and it felt both liberating, but equally scary. I recalled to Anton the following day how nervous I was and I'm not sure he understood. But if you're a woman and you can relate to this, then you know what I mean: "According to our study over a quarter of women (28%) feel anxious in a gym environment, and almost 61% would prefer to work out in a female-only space... A lack of knowledge around exercises and form... an overall sense of being uncomfortable... and feeling as though they're being stared at by other people... were top causes of gymtimidation for women."(hunkermoller.co.uk)

THAT section. THAT section where you hear the overexaggerated gasps, the colossal sounds of the crash of metal as dumbbells fly like lightning to the floor at the end of a set. THAT section where you observe the intimidating pump of biceps, combined with crimson faces in unison with amplified breaths. It showed that even despite the transformation of my body and my mind, my low self-esteem still manifested.

As time went by, my training split changed and I started doing three lower body sessions and one upper, merely because my upper body had a lot of muscle already: "The upper/lower split is very popular and allows you to spend more time on each muscle group while keeping your training frequency reasonably high... by alternating workouts for the upper and lower body, you get plenty of time for rest and recovery between training sessions." (Abelsson, 2022)

I hit my best numbers at that time (180kg on a hip thrust, 130kg on a deadlift and 80kg on a squat). I felt even more elated when men used to comment, men I didn't even know or had seen before. I would constantly get bombarded with questions like 'Are you a powerlifter?' and other comments about my strength. It felt amazing to be noticed and I could tell they were impressed. I got to the stage where I started to expect it. Even colleagues started to notice my physique changing and asked whether I was working out. I couldn't help my semi-humble smile when one colleague articulated; 'Yeah, I thought so, you look like you go the gym'. My confidence was growing every single month.

This was a milestone for me. I was once someone that had never picked up a dumbbell in my life, now I was becoming an intermediate.

My strength was soaring, yet, gradually putting on the pounds meant my clothes started to tighten and, in the end, I went up two dress sizes! The end of this bulking (or muscle-building phase as I like to call it now), didn't come without further embarrassment. My clothes were starting to feel so tight that coats were ripping under the armpits and my work blouses were uncomfortable, but I refused to buy bigger clothes.

One September afternoon while I was teaching a Year 9 class, I had an Incredible Hulk moment. Yes, an actual Incredible Hulk moment. It was the last lesson of the day, a lively class, my patience was wearing thin from the stressful day I'd had. The pupils had enraged me so much because of their volume, I raised my voice over theirs. I must have clenched my fists so tight because within a second, the button on the sleeve of my blouse shot off at the speed of light across the room. I was crying with laughter afterwards. One boy noticed it, but it was his shocked face and the rapid way his head spun in the direction of where the button flew, that really made me, and others hunch over uncontrollably as I retold this story later that evening in the gym. But everything I did, even if I wasn't confident, only caused me to reflect that just a bit further down the line, was a purpose and an end goal.

Two of my Instagram posts from that time really stand out when I think about how far I had come in a relatively short space of time, both physically and mentally. One in October 2018, whereby I had put four different pictures up (before weight training) and one that was taken towards the end of my first mini cut:

I'm not going to call this a "transformation" of aesthetics, mostly because I'm nowhere near where I want to be. These pics symbolise more the transformation of my attitude to food. I was the girl that tried EVERY diet under the sun: Weight Watchers, Dukan, 5:2, no carbs, Herbalife and other shake concoctions, skipping meals etc the list is endless! Exercise never involved weight training but relentless cardio. I'm proud to say that emotionally I have finally managed to achieve the balance and consistency but only because of the education I have gained due to @antonkostalas Seriously bro, you changed my life and I want to say thank you. I can honestly say (as cringe as this sounds!) I have never felt so happy. #weighttrainingforlife

As I reflect on what I wrote, I can see how completely transformed I was. I feel my sense of happiness and elation in the moment I was typing away on my old Samsung phone as I posted it. I think I was so shocked that the process was working as promised, given the number of years that I wasted to look different and feel different, having failed numerous times before. And, not to mention the relentless let downs from the fad diet industries. My attitude towards food and my habits started to change again.

Another post that stands out is a six-week progress picture of my abs. I was astounded that a mere six weeks into the diet, I saw abs for the first time in my whole life! I think just from these two posts, my confidence increased every day, and I began to have the balls to post my changing physique on social media. I did it for me and for the first time was putting ME first. *I was my only priority.*

There are so many females out there whose fear never diminishes. That fear of commitment and trust in someone to guide you, especially when it involves body image or bodyweight. So many women wouldn't dream of growing muscle and the inevitability of putting on some body fat. I didn't care.

Anyone who strives to knock your confidence or causes you to feel worthless, aren't worth knowing and their opinions not worth contemplating.

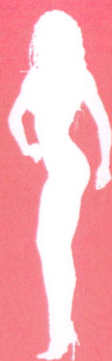

My clothes no longer fitted (at the end of the building phase I was 15lbs heavier) and it was difficult to accept, but I remember telling Anton I was not concerned how long it would take or how I would feel. I wanted to compete more than anything else. I'm pretty sure I avoided jeans altogether, simply because there was no chance of getting them past my knees! Yes, it was very hard being out of my comfort zone, especially as I'd already started posing classes at this size show day) and failed to imagine ever being lean. I didn't love my body, but every action had a purpose, so I kept looking forward.

An event occurred however, that knocked my confidence. Being at my biggest (but by no means obese), I recall walking down the street, and being summer I was wearing a sleeveless top. The sun was piercing, and I felt fully relaxed in the moment, as my strides kissed the pavement below my feet. A man walked past me, and, in that moment, shot down my flying positivity. He looked me up and down and started repeating with a look of disdain, 'Noooo, noooo'. In my head, all I could gather was his disapproval of my appearance and outward disgust about how I looked. In that second, I clammed up and the self-conscious feelings I already had of myself rose to the surface. In the next second, logic took over and I reminded myself why I was forcing myself to be uncomfortable. I just couldn't believe a stranger could express feelings of hostility to me with the audacity he did. No woman should be made to feel this way, certainly not by a stranger.

If anything like this has or does ever happen to you, don't pay any attention to what others think. What you want to achieve in your life is your prerogative and your priority. Anyone who strives to knock your confidence or causes you to feel worthless, aren't worth knowing and their opinions not worth contemplating. Although I am aware of this now, this recollection will always be one that stays with me. Even now I contemplate; was it really a negative reaction, or was it the result of my heightened sensitivity married with my low confidence? I'm still unsure.

The muscle-building phase was reaching its finale. I enjoyed the many cheat meals, the freedom of going out to eat, something I knew would be eliminated when I started the diet for stage.

I came to the realisation that my strength for this phase was far more important than aesthetics and I really felt the bee's knees when men continued to approach me and exclaim their shock at seeing a woman lift such heavy weights. I even accepted being more and more out of breath as my bodyweight increased but reminded myself of my look at the end. My last Instagram post of my bulking phase noted: *'An end to one phase and a start of another. Watch this space peeps.'*

Little did I know in just over five months later I would be in the best, leanest condition of my life, place in two categories, compete in a Fitness category which required more muscle mass and at the same time, embark on this prep journey alongside my brother and coach. I was ready to graft.

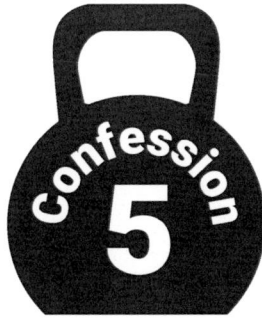

The Prep

*"All our dreams can come true if we have
the courage to pursue them."*
Walt Disney

To this day, I truly believe that no other prep will be as special as this one was in 2019. Most importantly, Anton and I were competing together and there are no words to describe how amazing this whole journey was, from start to finish. From the hardships and fears to the accomplishments and successes, regardless of the outcome, we were winners. As children we were inseparable, as adults even more so, but embarking on this fitness journey together, sharing our passion and love for training only solidified the strength of our whole relationship.

A week leading up to starting prep, Anton advised I take a week off training. This would enable my body to reset and rest until the prep commenced. I honestly didn't know what to do with myself that week. There is truth in that training gives you more energy. I had so much free time in the evening, yet I felt incredibly lazy and even more fatigued. For the first time, I didn't like how abstaining from training felt. And gosh do I remember that first leg session back with Anton the following Monday. Hands down, I have never felt so sick in my whole life. It was this first training session where I came to realise where that phrase "never skip leg day" came from.

In that first leg session, it was the front squats that did it. Every rest period I had, I quickly ran outside into the car park, hunching over on my hands and knees by the wall, trying to stop myself from vomiting. Others training in the studio at the time couldn't quite believe that my body was reacting in this way. All they ever saw was me giving it one hundred percent, and here I was again, feeling like a complete beginner and very unfit. After that, my body gradually got used to training again and I was starting to enjoy the process. I was surprised that even in just seven days of rest, my body found training an immense shock to the system.

It was only around this time that although I was still private on social media, I was becoming confident with posting more content. Every month I would send training footage videos to L and every month he would create a little prep update of what my training looked like. By this point, we had been together for two years and I was living in his flat in Hoddesdon, Hertfordshire. I was happy and everything in life was perfect. It was amazing to see the transformation in my body from these videos, month after month. Others on my Instagram were interested to watch and embark on my journey with me, through every session, every exercise, every rep.

I started writing and kept a prep diary. Journaling kept me focused; it was a fantastic release. It was a beautiful pink diary that had motivational quotes on every page. One by Junot Diaz really resonated with me: 'she would be a new person, she vowed. They said no matter how far a mule travels it can never come back a horse, but she would show them all.' It only made me even more determined to prove to others, but mostly myself, that I could completely transform, despite the number of years I had thought it impossible. Writing in this prep diary intensified my motivation.

As the weeks and months went by, I was enjoying the process much more as my body started to gradually change. In one session with Anton, I noticed my veins popping out of my arms, emerald, green rivers mapping themselves over my pale skin. I was completely shocked by this and others in the gym started to notice too. I questioned Anton: 'What is going on? Why are my veins popping out?!'

He enlightened me saying that's what happened the leaner someone became: "This process, known as filtration, causes a swelling and hardening of the muscle that is noticed during exercise. As a result of this swelling, cutaneous veins are pushed toward the skin surface, flatten to some extent, and appear to bulge. Such veins are more visible in persons with less subcutaneous fat." (Andrews, 2006) It seemed the strangest phenomenon to me. But finally, I looked like I trained for the first time in my life! I had become an athlete and I loved who I was becoming.

Be warned, there are always consequences to achieving a body like this. To my surprise, the first side effect only four weeks into the cut, was the loss of my menstrual cycle. I was not even super lean and could not believe that was the first thing to go, a sign that I had already reached my unhealthy body weight. There is a common misconception that it is just anorexic or bulimic females who suffer from this condition (Amenorrhea), because they have next to no bodyfat and are incredibly skinny. Hormones had changed before my own body, and it was only later on that I understood that this was the proper term for it: "Amenorrhoea is the absence of menstrual periods. Women who are elite athletes or who exercise a lot on a regular basis are at risk of developing athletic amenorrhoea. Exercise-related hormones and low levels of body fat are thought to affect how the sex hormones (oestrogen and progesterone) work". (Betterhealth)

I must confess, I enjoyed not having a cycle every month, not having to buy tampons, not worrying if I suddenly came on, the cramps or the hunger. I embraced it. Little did I realise how important this would be to me later, after the shows, when health and not aesthetics would become my priority.

Besides training and abiding by the macros I was given to an absolute T, (which I did over the whole prep), life carried on as normal. I was working in another school in Enfield as an Assistant Head of Key Stage Four. With less responsibility in this school, training and food were the focus in my life. I cannot say I particularly enjoyed the role; it was just a job for me that paid my bills and so unlike before, no emotional attachment or stress weighed me down.

The summer of 2019 was a great one and certainly a scorcher. By this time, L had legally divorced, and we had been together for two and a half years with a new addition; our jug Gurgi. This was something, back in 2015 I never believed would have ever happened. For so long his wife had refused and stalled the process, creating a seemingly endless limbo. Now, with the finalisation, we were free to be together without any lingering shadows. *He was fully mine*. Our relationship was something people could only dream of having or try and work to have. Yet, our love came so natural to each other, as natural as it was to breathe. Every morning, we would leave love notes for each other on multicoloured sticky notes on the kitchen counter. I missed him so much through the day and felt a rush of excitement upon parking outside our block when I came home and looked up towards the window; a heartwarming sight of his excited face and Gurgi's wagging tail. Their presence always made coming home feel like the best part of my day. I could never imagine a time where my love for him would end. And he was my number one cheerleader at this time.

I relished in the competing life; I didn't want it to take over completely. I still went on days out. Lots of coffee dates with L, days out with the family to Whitstable and Canterbury and had a great day with friends at Southend, going on the rides in Adventure Island. It was a great summer of that year. I made a vow to myself that I didn't want to become a complete hermit and let this prep run my whole life. Yes, I couldn't eat out with others, but I still attended birthdays, and with the utmost organisation and military precision, packed my meals in Tupperware. If we went out for drinks, I would opt for the sugar free options.

People misunderstand that when you follow macros accurately it is easier to cook meals yourself as you know *exactly* what is in them. Not many people realise all the added calories that go into, say, a piece of chicken. For example, adding oils or sauces can significantly increase the calories. These are all things everyday "normal" people rarely consider. But this was always in the forefront of my mind.

Most people in my circle were supportive. However, I would still be the receiver of negative comments like: 'You're boring', 'I feel sorry for you', 'Why are you doing this?' It was draining having to justify myself to others. Yet, I would remind myself that no one can really have an opinion on something they have never experienced themselves. Numerous occasions I questioned why my actions affected people this much, even more so what I chose to put in my mouth. While others enjoyed casual lunches and spontaneous treats, my diet often made me feel like an outsider. Social gatherings became a minefield of temptations and awkward explanations, deepening my sense of isolation as I adhered to my regimented routine.

When you are on a fitness journey such as this, you learn so much about the people closest to you, just as much as yourself. Their support is the only thing that really keeps you going, especially towards the end, when the end is *all* you can think about.

I was fourteen and a half weeks out and 9lbs down (weighing in at 133lbs) when I saw visible abs in the mirror. My body was transforming to an enormous degree and confidence was on the rise as people would continue to comment on how good I looked. I no longer felt bloated or sluggish like I did towards the end of my bulk. Admittedly, I was enjoying my meals, rotating my meats and vegetables around to avoid boredom and at the time I quite liked food prepping for the whole week on a Sunday (although it would take two hours!)

Despite not being starving, drinking sugar free sodas, squashes, and coffees, helped curb my hunger and made social situations more relaxing and enjoyable. I took pleasure in going for walks with Gurgi of an evening, especially if I felt hungry, but also to hit my steps. Steps were the only form of cardio I was doing at this point, as it burnt calories at a relatively low impact whilst at the same time, increasing my output.

Bodybuilders never tell you the extent to which food controls your mind and is the epitome of your whole existence. Watching food porn on Instagram or Facebook, wanting to smell other people's food becomes normal. Not to mention the dreams.

In one of my food dreams, I was ravenously eating a burger and chips, the barbecue sauce caressing my chin as my tongue glided across my mouth, then with the greatest satisfaction, licking my lips whilst swallowing a copious amount of mac 'n cheese. On waking, I could almost taste the thick gooeyness of the sauce and the heavenly smell of the hot cream of the velvety cheese in my mouth. It was enough to cause me to lick my lips as I sat up in bed that morning.

Food dominated my mind. It was on the highest pedestal and my whole being existed in its majesty. It was at the very top of my values and priorities.

In terms of exhaustion, I wasn't overly tired at this point, but the deeper into prep I became, the more conscious I was of my movement. At times I would become quite slow so I would have to remind myself to move more quickly or avoid leaning and sitting on things when all I was doing was standing. My body was trying to preserve as much energy as possible, as my calories got lower and lower. I did accept being slightly weaker and I recall on one of my Instagram posts outlining how I much preferred lifting heavy over aesthetics. Ironically, it became a chore to carry my new, lighter self.

As I became conscious of the side effects of mood swings, stress and anger, I did my best to ensure this didn't affect people around me. But this proved inevitable, in the last few weeks, even the calmest person can have the shortest fuse, and little things annoyed me about the people closest to me.

The whole process turned me into a super sensitive, irrational, neurotic person that I did not recognise.

As I became more sensitive, I tried to avoid getting anxious if I hadn't lost as much weight as I wanted in a week. Believe it or not, my whole world started to revolve around a number on a scale, which is not normal, but became habitual. I thought the worst about most day-to-day occurrences, even if it was a slight strain or pain in my muscles.

On one day, tears streamed uncontrollably during a session, merely because I felt a slight pain in my hip and instantly believed I would have to pull out of the shows. I became more dramatic, and every slight negative feeling blew up and was heightened beyond my control. Towards the end, my emotions got the better of me, even in sessions. At my most emotional, exercises such as front squats made me cry full on tears! Anton's reaction when he saw my eyes water, was to laugh, merely because the concept was so ridiculous. I was like a tap that could be turned on at any given moment. The whole process turned me into a super sensitive, irrational, neurotic person that I did not recognise.

I felt like an old, fragile granny going to bed at 9.30 p.m. every night, but I was so desperate for this recovery in addition to understanding how vital sleep and stress was for fat loss. I went as far as waking up at 4.50 a.m. in the morning if I had to train at 6.00 a.m. because I was working late or had parents' evening. The tunnel vision I had at the time was clear from what I had written at the end of one of my social media posts: 'I don't even care that I won't be eating cake on my 30th birthday'. Such a big sacrifice did not hinder the love I had for the process: 'having the best coach @antonkostalas and the support, encouragement and belief has confirmed this is worth it.'

I was loving even more how my body looked: veins popping, muscle definition, looking pumped especially after an upper body session, seeing full abs at 130lbs and feeling so good about myself, looking "toned." I was posting more and more physique photos on Instagram, and I was loving the attention I was getting, more because I just couldn't quite believe it was me when I looked in the mirror. I was feeding off it.

My 30th birthday was still memorable and not only because I couldn't indulge in cake! L and I stayed in Haworth, Yorkshire, a place that has always held a special place in my heart. For six years, it became an annual pilgrimage, and I didn't want to be anywhere else in the world.

We stayed in an Air BnB just because it was easier for me to stay on track, having full access to a kitchen, microwave and hob. However, the big hike to Top Withins (five miles in total) was a killer because I was at the stage of being about eight or nine weeks out and I would get tired more easily. Still, I didn't care that it was the first time in my life that I hadn't had cake on my birthday, all I envisioned every minute of the day were my poses and the stage.

As well as posting updated physique progress, I never failed to post the truths about competing and how I was feeling. Just over a month before the competition, I made a post with **"11 side effects that people would never be aware of while looking at my physique:**

1. *Hormones: haven't had a cycle since June and I was surprised they stopped so quickly.*

2. *Lack of concentration/memory: having to ask people to repeat basic instructions—I make small mistakes regularly like forgetting where I parked my car in the supermarket. I even have to label my Tupperware so I don't get my days mixed up.*

3. *Extreme tiredness: I have to stop for a few minutes even during a short walk—believe it or not this is worse than the hunger!*

4. *Physically weaker: I can't lift heavy at all compared to my bulk-this messes with your head and you feel like a beginner in the gym again.*

5. *Emotional during leg sessions: front squats have actually made me cry during 2 sessions*

6. *Experienced feeling 'zoned out' and people ask if you're ok because you are quieter than usual. You almost feel like a zombie or in a daze.*

7. *Looking at my watch constantly to countdown to the next meal*

8.   *Lack of patience with people and things that wouldn't annoy you before do now—often I'm good at hiding this*

9.   *Dreams about food: the other night I dreamt I indulged in Lindt chocolate and saw MyFitnessPal go into the minuses!*

10. *Development of bad eating habits: not leaving even a grain of rice on your plate so using your fingers to lick the plate (or even a dish that had chicken in from the oven because you want to eat every last morsel!)*

11. *Despite compliments from many people about how good/lean I look, no matter how much the scales tell you this too, you worry you may not be lean enough on stage".*

I wanted to enlighten others that I was more than just a lean physique. I felt at the time that people really needed to know the extent to which this sacrifice brought many negative effects on the body. It was not a normal way of life, nor a life to lead permanently. The thought of not having cake on my birthday now is something I cannot imagine, especially for a big one like a 30th or 40th!

Towards the end of the post, I reflected:

These are things that occur when you are prepping for a comp, but I am fully aware that this is a temporary extreme process. I go through this because as much as it is a physical test, it has taught me resilience, discipline, and mental strength I never knew I had. Being aware of the importance of recovery and balance after, I have been told, is so much more important and harder than the prep itself. Will Smith: "I will not be out-worked... if we get on that treadmill together... you're getting off first or I'm going to die."

It is amazing how one individual social media post can depict one moment in time. One moment in time to reflect an individual's success or failure, emotions, feelings or declarations, positive or negative. Like a diary entry that you are willing to share with others, that's what my Instagram became, even with only two hundred or so followers at the time. I had this irresistible urge to log and share every experience on Instagram as it happened. Each workout, meal and milestone became a snapshot, a story to broadcast. These constant updates made me feel connected, each post validating my journey and inspiring others along the way.

Will Smith:
"I will not be out-worked... if we get on that treadmill together... you're getting off first or I'm going to die."

To read over posts from that time is absolutely mind blowing. In all honesty, most of the prep didn't even feel like a diet and hands down it was only the last three to four weeks that were the worst, in terms of tiredness, hunger and a rollercoaster ride of emotions.

The pinnacle of my surprise was having to purchase size 4-6 clothes, and probably for the first time since I was aged twelve or thirteen! I had to buy a temporary wardrobe because I looked terrible in clothes; my size 10s would hang waywardly off my ultra-lean physique and even size 8s looked huge! Lack of libido was affecting my relationship, food and training were becoming the only thing I was immersed in and being a matter of weeks out when hunger and tiredness was at its peak, my brain was not functioning properly.

It was a typical autumn morning, not bitter cold, but not warm and comforting either. The sky was grey and glancing up at the trees, the foreboding impending winter was inevitable and fast approaching. Bare trees promised cold nights that were starting to draw in too soon, the golden leaves mourning the brightness of the scorching summer just passed.

As I wondered through Barclay Park with Gurgi, relentless shivers penetrated down my spine, a reminder of how lean I had become. As I looked down at the wet autumn leaves on the ground, thoughts of food echoed inside me once again and the dampness of the leaves from the rain reminded me of soggy cornflakes and warm creamy milk. The pang of hunger hit me again. I was shocked that something as defunct as fallen leaves, somehow still looked appealing and reminded me of food.

Other times I would park my car in a car park and forget where I had left it. How mad I was becoming; the cycle of these moments was exasperating. Talking about food and desserts was probably boring for many people around me yet said a lot about my obsession and want and need for it. It was the only time where my eyes would light up, there'd be a spark lit in me again and for those few moments I would feel "normal."

I recall L once admitting that the whole time I was on prep, the "spark" in me that he had known years prior, had disappeared. Overall, he was very supportive. But then again, I was always that strong-willed person that would always do what I wanted, even if that meant going against people's wishes. It is heart-breaking when the person you want to spend the rest of your life with points out a flaw and it hits you like a tonne of bricks and in a way, kills you inside. My behaviours nonetheless persisted. I had neither time nor patience to consider his needs. I was a horse with blinkers.

One night I spent the best part of an hour looking through Nigella Lawson recipe books, imagining all the things I would eat and bake after the shows were done. I even wrote a list of all the restaurants I would visit and all the foods I would indulge in. I was getting more and more excited for this process to be over and the mass consumption of food. It felt like an addiction, my drive was continuously sparked for me to complete this process.

Exciting things were happening as I was getting closer and closer to stepping on stage. I was asked by the gym studio I trained in with Anton to do a client testimonial with a videographer. It was such an amazing experience and something I had never done before. The mic was secured to my chest, and I was provided with questions about how training and dieting had changed my life. Afterwards, some footage was created showing me training with my new physique. I enjoyed every second and muttered to myself that this must be the sort of buzz a celebrity got when all eyes and cameras were on them. I didn't really know what to expect but was told I had done a really good job for someone who hadn't done it before. It was funny when we had to do a few takes with certain answers; I stumbled nervously over my words. The kind videographer guided me on how to construct my answers and then we would go on to do another take. In the moment I considered how much this process took away the realness of what we were trying to produce. Yet, the gym couldn't advertise a video such as this one with tons of mistakes! I felt like an actor with important parts being staged for better editing. It was relentless at times, but I honestly felt like a little celebrity.

Before I got too lean, Anton created my transformation video, and it got so many views when he uploaded it on Instagram. The video showed my physique six months prior to the present day. Nearly all viewers were those I had never met, especially as my brother had over 30k followers on this platform alone. I was not used to this attention at all, but it was really boosting my self-esteem, even though revealing my physique was probably the most invasive thing I'd ever done.

If I was tagged during training in Anton's stories, he would be overwhelmed with DMs from people commenting on how amazing I looked. I hadn't ever had this in my life, and I was smiling constantly. Everyone loves to be admired, and I was no different. Being so much leaner in posing lessons started to make things more real and I was so confident exhibiting my body, knowing I was so close to the end. I was proud to show it off at any given opportunity.

When we were two weeks out, Anton and I had a joint photoshoot booked with Simon Howard, a famous fitness photographer with all the top bodybuilders. I couldn't believe how long and tiring it was, I think it lasted about four hours! I enjoyed it so much and Simon made me feel so comfortable but holding poses and lifting weights for a posed shot was exhausting. My back was aching, the exhaustion was starting to hit me like a dive into water and my tedious breaths were the ultimate indication of how easily my energy could be sapped.

In between shots, Simon showed me a sneak peek on his camera of a photo he had taken of me facing the mirror. My instant response was complete disbelief and I cried out, 'That's not me!' as I laughed uncontrollably. I looked like something on the front of a health magazine.

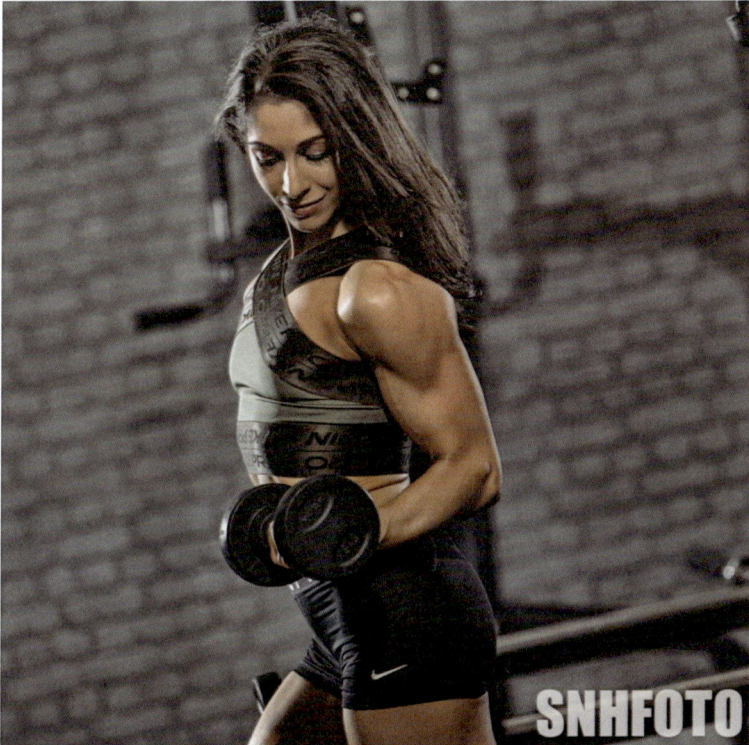

This busy day was probably the only day I didn't even think about food and how hungry I was and there was only one week left of this process. Posting these photos attracted over fifty likes! It still amazes me the photos that get the most likes on Instagram, but more on my opinion of social media later.

Two days before my show I posted my transformation, four photos wearing the same outfit at my heaviest 142lbs compared to my lowest weigh-in to date which was 114.65lbs, forty-eight hours before stepping on stage. The caption read:

If anyone told me 2 years ago that in 48 hours' time, I would be getting on stage showing my physique to 100s of people I would have laughed in their face!

142lbs:

- *Weight training was more enjoyable and I was at my strongest, hitting PBs in big compound lifts.*

- *Towards the end I felt like an overweight person training for the first time: out of breath constantly; sweating profusely, clothes not fitting due to the vast amount of weight and muscle I had deliberately put on*

- *Eating off meals 1-2 times a week was great socially and VERY enjoyable • Feeling full and never hungry before the next meal due to bigger portions*

- *NO ONE ever comments on your weight gain! Surprised?!?! (People did commend me on how heavy I could lift though!).*

114.65lbs:

- *Weight training slightly less enjoyable as hitting lower weights and so feel like a beginner in the gym as no real weight progression (despite the leaner physique!)*

- *Feel like a frail elderly person: out of breath and extreme tiredness even on short walks, cold ALL THE TIME (wearing hat, scarf and gloves even in 15 degree heat!) Clothes too big and having to buy new attire 3 sizes smaller (stage weight is not healthy or realistic!)*

- *Feeling hungry ALL THE TIME and never full after a meal—did I already mention getting down to stage weight is not healthy or realistic?! Worth noting: I have enjoyed all my foods on the cut, just wish they were bigger portions!!*

- *EVERYONE comments on my leaner body in a positive way.*

Do I regret either? No. Yes. They are 2 extremes but without being bigger and stronger before, I would never have been able to get as lean as I am now for stage.

MOST IMPORTANTLY: I want to be healthy and in the middle of these pics (roughly 125-130 pounds), still having an off meal once or twice a week and building up even more muscle this year! I will NEVER stop training because I LOVE IT! RECOVERY for me after these comps will be an even bigger challenge for me—even more so important than these phases!

I looked so ill at my leanest, but it's mad to think on stage I looked huge. I looked like a skeleton in normal clothes. Secondly, I'm laughing to myself; I genuinely thought I could maintain my ideal weight. It upsets me to think how much this process changed me in a negative way, indefinitely. As much recovery will always be very similar to a recovering addict of any kind, my relationship with food in this case never went back to how it was and altered forever. I learned to manage it, deal with it and accept it.

In the last few weeks and days leading up to the show, I was elated and excited knowing I was so close to the end, imagining all the treats I would indulge in. But also, other more anxious thoughts filled my head; a rush of fear of something going wrong on the day, my heel breaking on stage, or something worse happening like having a serious injury or being hospitalised due to an accident, or someone close to me dying on the day. All irrational thoughts of course.

Something did happen to me but thankfully I was OK. One morning walking Gurgi before work, I fell down a slippery flight of stairs in the block of our flat and fell with force flat on my back. My initial reaction was panic that after all this sacrifice I wouldn't be able to get on stage. Thankfully I came away with just a few bruises, but because the walk was fasted, as soon as I lifted myself off the stairs, a horrible headache hit me, and a rush of sickness overwhelmed me as bile rose to my throat and I was hunched over waiting for the sick to leave my body. My body, deprived of its usual vitality, struggled to keep up, highlighting the toll that my rigid regimen was taking on me.

At my leanest leading up to peak week, the reactions from family and friends couldn't have been more opposite. In the gym when I was pumped, I would get comments like, 'Wow, your body is amazing.'

'You look so good.'

and from mainly family members attending functions, I would get snake-slaying comments like,

'What's happened to your face?'

'You are skinny.'

'You've lost so much weight.'

'Your face looks gaunt.'

You can't please everyone; and that goes for every aspect of life. My advice to you, just please yourself.

Peak week (the last seven days leading to the show) was not as scary as I thought it might be, or how it's generally viewed to be: "During this week the athletes' goals are to focus on increasing the intermuscular lipid stores as well as their intermuscular glycogen stores, with careful consideration regarding the concentration of water in their muscles, to ensure they look the fullest they can on stage while still maintaining a conditioned look." (2022, blogs.brighton) In all honesty it was the easiest week compared to the last two years. Despite being at my lowest calories (1100) for two of the days it was the easiest; training was different. Compound exercises (the main lifts e.g.: squats, deadlifts and bench presses) were taken out and more "squeezy" stuff was put in. High reps using lighter weights on things like cable flyes, kickbacks were incorporated. It felt easy too knowing I was one week away, so my motivation was at its highest during this time and there was no time left for any fuckups.

The strangest part of all was the water loading. I was drinking seven litres of water a day, Monday through to Friday and on Saturday, the day of the show, I had to cut out water the night before and only take little sips on the Saturday. You can imagine how much I was running to the toilet the entire week! I was so depleted I remember trying to pull my skin but there was nothing to pull, it looked more like an elastic band. My fingers and toes and hands looked so skinny, my rings hung loose, it was the strangest thing I've ever experienced. On top of all of this, I also had to bear the brunt of thirty minutes cardio with every session and thirty minutes of posing which I had to do every day leading up to the show.

Carb loading (consuming a significant increase in carbohydrates) on the Friday was great though but what was even weirder in terms of my meals, was the fact that I had to cut out vegetables and fruit because of the bloating it would cause. Salt was kept the same though a lot of people assume you should cut it out. The key was to just keep it consistent to avoid any massive fluctuations in my bodyweight. Also, I took vitamin C tablets three times a day to ensure my body fought possible illnesses; my immunity was at its lowest during this time.

I drove to get my first lot of tan the night before. Standing completely buck naked in line with other women while trying to control my shivers was unbearable. On the one hand, no one is self-conscious about being naked because your body is at its peak of perfection yet feeling you could die from frostbite made me want it to be over. Whilst standing in line, I couldn't help but be struck by the eerie resemblance to the haunting images of people in Auschwitz. The vulnerability, the exposed skin, the skinny arms enlaced around their emaciated bodies. The quiet, orderly queue brought this uncomfortable and sombre comparison to mind; a stark opposition of how we would all portray ourselves to be later in the day.

After it was done, I had to be so careful to avoid smudging it. I had to sprint out of the building with my umbrella that day wearing flip flops and a tracksuit to avoid the puddles and the possibility of streaks. That night my bed sheets were permanently stained, not to mention the complaints I got from L about the toilet seat changing colour!

I got an early night but was buzzing with excitement going over my routine about three or four times in my head thinking when I wake up, the day I've been waiting for, will have finally arrived. The end was in sight.

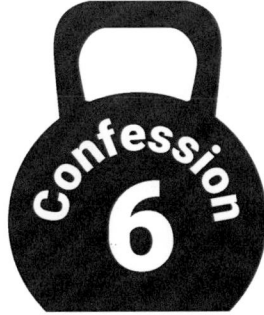

Changing Careers

"Everyone thinks of changing the world,
but no one thinks of changing himself."
Leo Tolstoy

Before I go into the real-life experience of show day, it is probably important to rewind a little bit to about four weeks or so before the show where I made the most life changing decision to give up a life, a job, a passion and endure a 360-degree life turn almost overnight.

I'd been at the school in Enfield for nearly two years where I was a main English teacher and an Assistant Head of Key Stage 4. I was starting to get frustrated. As lovely as the department was, they had been teaching there for over ten years and were more willing to continue to put up with all the politics. All I could see was how their constant pessimism affected the atmosphere in the office. Their daily complaints and grumblings reminded me of how Anton used to point out my own negative tendencies. It was a poignant reminder of someone I once was, but for the first time, my eyes were open to the person I truly wanted to be.

Given my traumatic experience in the school I was working at before in Essex whereby I was one of over fifteen people bullied by the deputy head teacher and decided to report her to the Governors when I left, in addition to the stress and mental health issues I developed from being a Head of English before that, I became so strong I learnt to stop caring what others thought of me. I wasn't going to put up with any more shit from people.

This is what training does, it makes you put yourself first and consider your own needs above anything else. You may call it selfishness; I call it self-care and self-love.

I was annoyed that even though I was in my second academic year there, I was still on a fixed term contract. I thought I had done more than prove myself. I never had any behaviour issues in my classes, I was always on time for every deadline, I would plan lessons to the best of my ability and make them as fun and as enjoyable as possible and would receive good feedback on my lesson observations. The truth is, despite how hardworking I was, I felt unappreciated and undervalued. I was a great teacher and yet I could not believe that despite my requests to be put on a permanent contract to guarantee a safety net, I was told that I would have to spend another year on a fixed term because my own Head of Department was on a fixed term and money was very tight for the school: "Early data from the National Association of Head Teachers... shows that 50% of heads say their school will be in a deficit...This comes as Jeremy Hunt has made clear that all departments, including education, will be expected to make cuts as part of the government's debt reduction plan... most schools having to lose essential teaching and support staff." (Fazackerley 2022)

The new Head teacher (not the one that employed me initially) had already started causing a stir; he initiated financial cuts by making many staff members redundant. Additionally, those in higher positions like Heads of departments had their workload tripled and therefore had to oversee more members of staff. Looking back, it was easy to hate him; at the time his decisions seemed callous and unfair, he was another slave to the regime, forced to implement policies beyond his control, but I wanted no part of it.

I started to loathe the way schools were being run. It made me realise that every new school I ever started at was always that little bit worse than the previous and more and more of them were not considering the students as a priority. It made my blood boil.

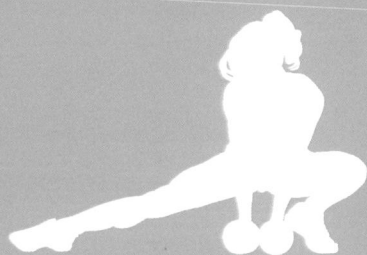

This is what training does, it makes you put yourself first and consider your own needs above anything else.

Having been in education for over ten years, I believe it safe to say that schools are now run as businesses, they are not in any way there to serve the students' needs (or rather students' needs are never the priority). Teachers are treated worse than any other, especially those with the least responsibility. I saw so much injustice yet could do nothing about it. Staff being mistreated, unfair goals being set for them in terms of exam results, the damage to their physical and mental health which I could only see spiral into an oblivion. No one cares and last of all, you are kept in your place. No matter how unfair a decision, those staff that would question decisions, would only be seen to be undermining your superiors.

At this point, six or seven weeks away from my show, I knew I had to fill in a leave of absence form. Because of all the "time off" you get as a teacher unless you are off sick (and even then, if you are vomiting your guts up you still must plan your lessons and email them in as cover for the cover supervisor) you are not allowed to take any leave. You may be lucky to get part of a day off to attend a funeral and some head teachers ensure that it is unpaid.

When I put the request in, I felt confident that I would be allowed one Monday off (the day after the show) because I had a photoshoot in Wales that day. My own head of department was allowed a Monday off to nurse his hangover after a Sunday wedding and another colleague in my department was allowed another few days off after a half term holiday to travel back from a christening abroad. So, what was I worried about?

A few days passed and I still hadn't received authorisation, paid or otherwise. When the email came through eventually, I could not believe that instead of a rejection or at least unpaid leave, a short, blunt email informed me that the Head Teacher wished to discuss my request in person. I was taken aback. I had to face him and justify it.

I knocked nervously on his door three times and heard his bellowing yes to enter. I felt like a student rather than a member of staff. He asked me to sit down and as I did there was a very long awkward silence. In my head I was wondering why on earth this guy wasn't starting the conversation if he was the one requesting to see me. I thought my written request was self-explanatory. With a little bit of bravery within me, I eventually broke the silence and posed the question: 'You wanted to see me about my leave of absence request?' He said yes, he wanted to know what it was for. Again, in my head I kept thinking, does this guy not read anything he is given? I thought it was self-explanatory; I had written down: 'to take part in a bodybuilding show'. So, when I explained the situation, he looked very confused and dumbfounded. He kept repeating the question: 'You're going to be in a bodybuilding show?' at least three times and at least three times my reply maintained, 'Yes… yes…'

By the look on his face, I could have told him I was taking part in the Olympics, it was one of disbelief, humour and confusion. I did explain that I hadn't any Year 11 classes that day (and that it was only one day) and that my colleagues in the department had already said they wouldn't mind covering my three lessons. Instead of praise or shock or disbelief that I would be doing something that not many people could say that they have done, he said in an extremely short and abrupt manner, 'So what am I supposed to say to the governors? That you want time off for one of your *personal hobbies?*'

The realisation hit me as to how weak I was and even the desperation in my voice was embarrassing when I begged, 'What if it was unpaid?' He then replied sternly, 'I will get back to you within 48 hours.' His domination shattered me. I felt completely broken. If I could imagine being the observer in this room, I envisioned myself like broken glass at the slightest touch. Shattered beyond repair.

Desperate to leave his office as soon as possible, I exited through his door shaking with rage. Walking as quickly as I could down the corridor and up the stairs, I burst into tears, out of embarrassment, humiliation, and anger at my own weak nature. He made me feel worthless, undervalued, and disempowered. He proved to be yet another narcissist head teacher like many others in power. I couldn't wait to leave the building. In fact, I began to notice on most days I would be staring at the clock wondering if it was after 4.00 p.m. so I could head to the gym. I didn't want to be here anymore.

The only thing I became excited about during the working week was my session with Anton. Getting through this prep was the only thing I had tunnel vision for and NOTHING and NO ONE was going to stand in my way, not even the person who ran the place.

After wiping the tears away hastily from my face, I walked through the door of the English office, my colleagues in anticipation asking immediately how it went, what I was going to do. Sadly, there were only two options; either pull out of the shows or pull a sickie for that day and face a disciplinary. A disciplinary would mean it staying on my record forevermore, it would mean a bad reference if I left, and it could mean that it would make my life hell if I chose to stay. Staying meant being stuck in a cycle of frustration and routine, but leaving offered the promise of freedom. The dilemma, a tornado in my head, was paralysing. Each choice carried its own set of risks, leaving me torn between security or the hope of something better. I wanted better. I wanted more.

I knew at that moment I needed to leave teaching behind. I knew I would never quit what I had worked years in the gym for and all I could think about was how to work around this. Little did my colleagues know, of course I was going to go off sick, but it would be indefinitely. The fact that I was taken for a ride with my contract, not being made permanent for over a year and the person who I worked for in the utmost position of power to crush my dreams, were enough reasons that I was done with this school, done with the regime, done with the system, and done with teaching.

I broke down in tears again at the start of my session with Anton that same day when I told him what had happened. Without thinking and without hesitation I said to him, 'I want to leave teaching. I don't want to do it anymore and I want to do what you are doing'. The biggest smile came across his face and all he replied was 'I know... I know,' nodding his head in agreement. He overwhelmed me with the amount of confidence he had in me. He then told me the most beautiful words that gave me the ultimate relief and confirmed my decision. 'So, the studio is expanding, and they are opening another gym. They are going to need more PTs.' I couldn't believe my ears. In that split second, I pictured my future. Me and Anton, working together, but also me living my dream of being in a gym every day and doing what I love, what I was passionate about. I was ecstatic and, in that moment, I felt a huge burden being lifted off my shoulders. He then went on to tell me that he knew the company I could use to get qualified in as little as eight weeks!

I knew my calling and I knew this was it.

The very next day instead of being sad and gutted about how I was being treated, I used that energy to plan. I was going to call the company to see when I could get enrolled, and I already knew that I would leave the school and go off sick long before my competition date. No one was going to crush me again or spoil my dreams.

I was sat idly in a free period thinking about how I was going to get out of this, a pile of Year 11 exam papers sat at my desk, the words making no sense in my head, so dropping my red pen confidently on the desk I opened a blank word document on my laptop and started to type.

The words in my head magically appeared on the screen and I kept going until everything was released. This was the piece that was not only a mere glimpse into my new future, but the start of the next chapter of my life. Writing this, only confirmed the path I was going to take. I titled it "My Epiphany" and I went on to send it to Anton, my mum and my best friend:

Once upon a time nearly ten years ago, my twenty-year-old self wanted nothing more than to change young people's lives; to improve them, to help them develop life skills, morals, to love literature, to improve their literacy, to work well with others and develop social skills, to respect and appreciate me as their educator. I used to feel that amazing buzz; that buzz where you feel like your stomach is turning inside out, where you develop relationships with students that forever remain in your memory-when you teach those lessons that either make them laugh, or cry. I remember my eight or nine-year old self, lining up all my toys in rows or a circle, reading out a register, recording my lessons over an old-fashioned tape recorder, or writing numbers or letters on a blackboard. All I ever wanted to do was to teach-to live, breathe, dream it.

I remember working for two weeks at Mount Grace School just before I started university, sitting in various lessons writing comments in my exercise books such as "this is all I want to be" and "I can imagine doing it". I felt that immediate love come over me, especially when I had interactions with those students.

The first few years of teaching were the best. I remember telling people that 'It's not a job but a lifestyle', not caring if I worked twelve- or thirteen-hour days or how long it took me to plan lessons because it was me, my identity. I never felt a love, passion or enthusiasm for anything like that before. Getting promoted built my confidence and made me feel that I knew who I was.

TTA—my first school. Your first school is like your first love-you never forget it or the impact it had on your life, and nothing compares to it. Those kids I have never forgotten, no others have compared to them, and it made me who I was.

My love for teaching died four years ago when I became a Head of English. Money, being a boss, making decisions was not worth the lack of life or the detriment of my health. After that, being bullied by people in power, struggling with changes in a curriculum, getting fed up with the politics and the constant reinventions or cycles of how to teach and "improving teaching and learning" either made me grow up, wake up or was it just a realisation that I never knew before, being a young, inexperienced NQT.

I had an epiphany over the weekend. Maybe it's because I was told doing a show would make me realise things about myself, things about others or make you realise what you want in life. All I know is that I have been unhappy in this career for 4 years and let each year slip by, *survive each day, hoping that the next school would be better than the previous. All I have gained is disappointment after disappointment— heads and senior management that continue to bully, show lack of respect and support, make you jump through impossible hoops of fire, make you feel you're never good enough or "you could have also done this or this". I used to frown upon older teachers when I first started out when I was surrounded by negativity. My instant reaction was "I don't know why they don't just quit teaching". I always said to myself that if I felt like that, I must do something to change it.*

The truth is the love and enthusiasm that I had has died. It no longer exists. Every day I wake up, stand in front of hundreds of students and know that deep down I am living a complete lie. I am going along with something I don't believe in. A social media post written by a female bodybuilder last week said, "There's no point wasting your time doing something you don't believe in". That hit me HARD. It made me reevaluate what I want in life. It made me realise that it's not about the school politics, it's not even about the ways of testing (again which I don't agree with), it's about fighting the whole government education system—which will never happen. Do I believe we should be teaching Shakespeare to students in 2019? No. Do I believe we should be killing literature for them by making them memorise hundreds of quotes? No. I loved Shakespeare aged 11. My mother took me to watch 'Macbeth' at the theatre and I loved it. I loved it because I wasn't forced to read it back-to-back, wasn't forced to memorise hundreds of quotes or write what language or structural technique was in it. I am disgusted that this whole education system has let ME down. I don't agree with it, nor do I believe in it anymore.

When I look at the clock at 3.20, I anticipate leaving work to go to the gym. When I am in there, I feel alive, I feel that buzz that I used to feel, if not even stronger. I appreciate the progress I have made, the positive comments by others who have also seen this, how it's changed my mindset, how it's made me a positive person, how it has saved my life. I want to help others do this. I know it's going to be hard-time wise, financially etc., etc., but I want nothing more than to learn. I want to be the best. I want to change people's lives in terms of health—physically, mentally and their overall wellbeing. Being in a gym I feel ME. I feel it's a new goal—after the sadness I will feel when the shows are over, I feel that I have a new purpose.

The negative people around me remind me of the importance of security, of holidays or working hard to be where I got to. The truth is, I have given teaching a decade of my life. I don't regret it. I feel I can't carry on coasting in a job I know I'm unhappy with. It's not even about the "type" of schools that I have been to, it's bigger. I don't believe nor have faith in this system anymore. This feeling I have seems to get stronger and stronger every day. I envision myself doing client check-ins instead of marking books, teaching adults the techniques on how to squat instead of teaching them Dickens' quotes, solving or suspecting an injury—instead of suspecting a learning need in a child, telling off a client for not progressing (as opposed to telling off a child for stupidity). I envision it so much. I want it so much that I feel there is nothing else I want, I will die if I don't try.

Again, regardless of starting again at the age of 30, financial changes, lack of holidays, I KNOW this is the right step to take and I KNOW I will succeed. It is scary as I have never left schools, never known anything else, always knew what I wanted, and it was always clear who I was or who I was going to be. This feeling right now of being a little lost is unnerving. But I feel I have felt these feelings and coasted along for too long without doing something about it: 'There is no point wasting your time with doing something you don't believe in.'

PROS OF STAYING:

- *Holidays—good for future children*
- *Financial security*
- *It's familiar*
- *Enjoy working with students*

CONS OF STAYING:

- *Feeling unhappy in my career—Feel lethargic about going in*
- *No sense of fulfilment anymore—lack of enthusiasm*
- *Don't like the politics*

- *Don't like stress of results*
- *Treatment of staff*
- *Constant monitoring*
- *Marking*
- *Admin overload-data drops, seating plans*
- *Don't agree with what I'm teaching—feeling I'm living a lie-don't enjoy teaching Shakespeare etc., just for exam*
- *Have to look for another job anyway-contract ends August 31st, 2020*

Emotion encompasses me as I read this over. It still stands to be the scariest, but the best decision I ever made. I had my plan. Once I spoke to the guy in charge of training aspiring PTs to get qualified, he said that it would not only be government funded, but that I could start the day after my first show. Without hesitation, I signed up. Now all I had to do was book an appointment with the doctor to sign me off sick to ensure I still got paid and plan when I was going to do it.

I'm pretty sure it was merely two or three weeks at most since the meeting with the Head teacher where I knew my time was up. The last grain of sand from the hourglass had fallen. I went about my day, complete poker face, still doing my job, marking my Year 11 exam papers, even though I wouldn't be seeing them through, knowing I was a step closer to leaving. For the first time in my life, I did not feel guilty because I knew I was more important.

Then, that epiphany: I WAS MORE IMPORTANT.

On my last morning, I drove through the green iron gates thinking whatever happens, I'm never going to do this again. Carrying my bags lethargically from the car and walking nervously up the two flights of stairs knowing this would be my last day in this school, in teaching.

My head of department bumped into me on my way in and attempted to engage in casual conversation, enquiring whether I was going to go for the line manager's job, because she was also leaving because of discontent. His smile and unexpected warmth caught me off guard, but eased the tension I felt in myself, knowing the effect of what I was going to do would have on him in the months to follow. Repeatedly, he said, "You would be so good for it" and that he'd be delighted if I did. I could tell he was massaging my ego, enquiring out of pure desperation to fill the position. He knew I was the next one in line to take on that position. The rhythm of our steps mirrored each other as we navigated the familiarity but silence of the corridor, absent of the loud bustles of students which would be rife within the next hour.

As we continued to walk, I stared at the white walls that now seemed cold and uninviting. Their stark emptiness reflected the sterile atmosphere of the building, devoid of warmth and personality. I knew if I chose to stay, I'd become exactly like those white walls; scuffed, bland and invisible. I simply replied, 'No, I've done my time.' Little did he know the true irony of those words. I think that day was a Tuesday, and my plan was to keep calling in sick for the next couple of days and then book an appointment with my GP.

3.30 p.m.

I stared at the hands on the clock anticipating this exact moment. I muttered under my breath, 'Wow Tash, this is it. The start of your new life.'

Slowly, I packed my bag as normal, sneakily putting the last few bits of my personal stationery and belongings inside. Taking one last look at my classroom, my hand caressed my desk for the last time, and I placed my school ID lanyard in the top drawer. Glancing around the room, ghostly memories filled my head; sounds of the students' voices, loud chatter and excitement, the wind cascading from the nearby open window and the sounds of the turning pages of their exercise books, all of which I would never hear again. The stale, musty yet familiar smell lingered in the air, a testament to its long history. I observed the chipping paint on the walls, the desks with layers of graffiti, the marks of countless students that had sat in front of me. The room looked bare and haunting, the atmosphere felt tired, as if the room itself had absorbed the years of weariness that I had felt in this career. For the first time, I noticed the profound silence of my classroom. This stillness struck me with a sombre resonance, reminiscent of a funeral or a remembrance ceremony: 'Here lies Miss Kostalas, beloved teacher and an inspiring example to us all, forever in our hearts.' As I let out a huge sigh of relief, I closed the door behind me.

I walked confidently out the escape exit (even though on numerous occasions we were berated for this in staff meetings) and I remember taking a big deep breath in and out as I walked to my car. No one saw me and no one was any the wiser. It was my own little secret. After placing my belongings in the boot of my car, I stood and stared at the grand building, feeling a wave of relief wash over me. The structure, once looming and oppressive, now seemed insignificant in the grander scheme of what life might hold for me. As I sat in the car, putting on my seatbelt, I drove out of the car park and whispered goodbye under my breath. As I crawled out of the overpowering green metal gates, I never looked back, a lightness coming over me; I was finally free.

Take heed. If you are still carrying on with something that you know that deep down makes you unhappy—whether it be the relationship you're in, the job you're in, an estranged relationship with a family member or friend, just know your worth. Don't carry on. You're the most important person, so do something about it.

To you V** *********y. Thank you. Thank you for treating me like shit that day. If it wasn't for your narcissistic attitude, your detestable behaviour, your insufferable leadership, your vile actions towards others, I never would have taken the plunge. I am so happy we had that encounter that day. If not, I dread to think what other hoops of fire I would be jumping through now to massage your ego, or make you look good for the school. I hope you know that you were the last person I ever allowed to treat me in that way. Thanks for altering my future for the better and thanks for reminding me that it is people like you, bullies like you and J**** R********n that have made me a better person and tore me away from the revolting institution that is now "education" for you to control and revel in.

Once, I thought you both had the ultimate power, that your high position signified ultimate success. Now, I have come to realise your power was just an illusion, a magic trick and in fact, me having more control of my life now, being my own boss and not being a slave to the system that controls *your* life, has brought me peace. I believe if you are someone that goes through life mistreating people, you will never be truly happy or at peace in your life.

I'm not a bitter person. Believe it or not, despite how I feel about people in teaching who have bullied, criticised, disempowered me, made me feel weak, vulnerable, and worthless. I am not someone that holds a grudge against anyone.

I don't HATE.

I DESPISE unjustified treatment of others, good people. I count myself as one of the lucky ones. Lucky because I am one of the many people that have left teaching because I didn't want to be set up to fail anymore. [1]I can never forget how I allowed people to treat me, and it has been a massive lesson learnt. I have learnt not to *need* that system. It's also worth noting, that every single person I know who has left teaching, has NEVER returned. What does that tell you?

***

I managed to complete my PT course in four weeks. In a way, it extended the hype as I started two days after my first show and two weeks later I was doing my second, so I got a lot of respect from others in the class. My tutor was lovely, the people in the class were just fresh out of school so it was annoying seeing such stupid childish behaviours like turning up an hour late with headphones in, chatting while the tutor was trying to talk. But I'm glad I got it done. I did know more than half the people in the class in terms of training and nutrition. I already felt confident being two steps ahead of them.

It still grinds on me how easy it is to become a PT today. There are

---

1   44% of England's state school teachers plan to quit by 2027. Over half (52% of teachers say their workload is either 'unmanageable or 'unmanageable most of the time' , up from 35% in 2021 – (neu.org.ukpress-releases/state-education-profession

so many shit PTs out there and to be honest, PTs get a bad rep-and rightly so! There are so many that don't deal with client's nutrition or practise what they preach or make their clients accountable or manage to get their clients to where they want to be. I don't know how they can take people's money. I was shocked walking through the park once when I saw a PT training a woman who was squatting with such bad form that I nearly wanted to intervene! She was leaning over so much her head was nearly on the ground!

Anyway, I regress. This was the post I wrote when I finally got qualified. I had escaped teaching, I had placed in two categories in my shows, and I was embracing my new life; once a client, now turned coach:

George Eliot: "It is never too late to be what you might have been".

I've kept this quiet for a while but after ten years of being a Secondary School English teacher, I finally took the leap of faith and am finally doing what I'm passionate about, what I love and believe in.

Truth: my love for teaching died four years ago but I carried on coasting like many do.

Truth: weight training tested my limits and competing in 2 shows gave me courage to make this decision. Someone once said that if I accomplished that I would feel invincible and would feel I could do anything.

It happened. Now I don't know what I was afraid of.

Take it from me: there is no point wasting your time doing something you don't believe in. B********, you gave me wings (HEART)

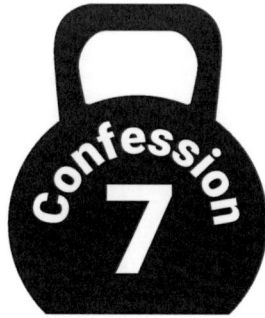

The Shows

"To be a champion, compete; to be a great champion, compete with the best; but to be the greatest champion, compete with yourself."
Matshona Dhliwayo

If you ask most women what the best day of their lives are, they may say: 'The day I got engaged', 'The day I got married', 'The day my baby was born.' Although ordinary yet extraordinary experiences which I have not yet experienced, competing is the closest I have ever been to feeling similar emotions on the same level as these life milestones. The hype, experience and gratification are something no one will be able to replicate and true understanding is the outcome from the experience itself.

The hype is unreal, the way your stomach does a thousand somersaults over and over as you wait for your category to be called. The day before the show, all athletes are required to sit in a meeting where the host outlines the timings of the day, what your T walk (your routine) should look like and other general pieces of information, so everyone feels comfortable on the day.

Anton and I sat excitedly, me hanging off the chair with ants in my pants thinking to myself that this was happening, that I got here. What once felt like years away, would in the next twenty-four hours disappear in the blink of an eye.

Waiting around backstage is probably the most relentless part of the day. Glancing across the rooms and spaces, tanned bodies are everywhere, half naked bodies prancing around, people lying on the floor with their legs up in the air (we didn't do this but some people do, something to do with blood flow I believe). People you do interact with share stories of their prep or tell each other what they will eat as soon as the night is over. You meet some amazing people and engage in some interesting conversations with others backstage regarding their individual fitness journeys, experiences, and backgrounds. Despite our different paths, the camaraderie and mutual respect amongst competitors, forged through our shared passion and dedication for the stage, made this day unforgettable.

Show day is meant to be the most exciting day of the whole process. Yet, what I found surprising is the amount of people that lose that trait of humbleness; something which at some point everyone has, but somehow gets lost along the way. Some of the bikini girls that day came across as bitchy, arrogant and superior. Because the changing rooms are unisex and you must share them with anyone, Anton and I took one room. Little did we know it was filled with screaming big-boobed blondes (fake of course). As we entered lugging our suitcases behind us, their eyes met Anton's, and one pulled a strop and announced loudly, 'No we don't want boys in here.' I literally couldn't believe her hostility. One of the friends of this cow apologised. Withholding our anger, Anton and I stormed into another extremely tiny room, on my way out whispering under my breath, 'Arseholes.'

Although a dark, cramped and dingy room with no window and no space at all except for one mirror, one shelf and one chair, we ended up sharing it with two more mature ladies who were lovely. One thing I noticed that day was that the older competitors were the nicest of them all. You can tell that their maturity and life experiences made them less showy, less arrogant, humbler and I was so thankful to have these two women with us, even though I was up against one of them in one of my categories.

Timing is everything. Food is everything on show day too. As you are drinking merely a couple of sips throughout the day to stay dehydrated, you have to ensure you time your carb loading properly, maybe an hour before you step on stage, in order for your muscles to fill out beforehand. I think Anton and I were munching on jam and rice cakes, others around us were indulging in huge chocolate bars, melted chocolate smears outlining the rims of their lips, which looked more like a binging session than a planned muscle pump. In our second show, Anton and I wolfed down one and a half Krispy Kreme doughnuts. You can imagine how much our taste buds had been sparked as we licked the icing lovingly from our fingers and around the base of our mouths.

Despite eating and sipping on water, we were so cold. Our entire bodies quivered with every hour that passed. I didn't take my coat off until I was ready to go on stage: "Related to adaptive thermogenesis, and low bodyfat levels. Fat is an insulator, it keeps heat in the body, however as you drop fat and energy intake, your body adapts to save energy, you stop fidgeting as much and shivering as much. Combine this with the fact you've probably shaved off a lot of your body hair and you just get cold. This phenomenon was first reported in people suffering from starvation, and hunger strike. As soon as the calories and the bodyfat comes back athletes stop feeling the chill." (Chappell, 2022)

The waiting around was boring and tiring and because we were dehydrated, we didn't feel our best. Headaches came and went on the day, but the adrenaline caused us to ignore the pounding in our heads.

You step on stage feeling zombie-like, your brain in a haze, your gait like those of a stumbling drunk. That backstage feeling kicks in when your category is called. And even though still a very long wait before you go on stage, your mind and heart are racing. You're constantly going over your routine in your head, envisioning it on stage and you feel your heart pounding louder and louder, in sync to the deafening booms of the music. Also, the other thing to think about is that you are pumping your muscles before stage shortly after your carb load. Again, something else which is necessary to look your best on stage but looks completely unconventional and comical all at the same time.

I think I may have lost about three or four bands backstage when I competed, like food, everyone wants it in their hands. Things like band openers, kickbacks to pump your glutes, squats and press-ups are done repeatedly for three to four sets even as you are waiting in line. It is like a workout before you go on stage to complete your routine. When you're cold, hungry, tired and nervous all at once, it feels even tougher and even more relentless!

Waiting in line backstage is the most nerve-racking experience. A memory of entering the hall of my first GCSE exam is the closest I can relate it to; the thumping of my heart, hands shaking rapidly, becoming clammy with nervous sweat. All you can hear are the crowds and the music, but all you can focus on is you. For Miami Pro, my first show, I signed up for three categories (Bikini, Wellness and Fitness) and it was only until I was in line with the Bikini girls that I knew I was in the wrong category, and funnily enough it was the only one I didn't place in. But, after needing to go on stage another two times and to do my routine again I didn't let it put me off. I felt even more confident with every step I took in those heels on that stage.

Just before my number was called, my hands were trembling and my heart was beating rapidly. I couldn't believe this was the moment I had waited two whole years for. Everything was worth it, whatever the outcome.

"Number 130, Miss Natasha Kostalas!"

As soon as I stepped on the X, the bright lights hit me and all I could do was ignore the screams from the audience. I just kept imagining I was back in the studio with my posing coach, that's all I was willing to focus on, to diminish the nerves that were taking over. I remembered to keep giving the judges eye contact as well as the photographer, another thing that was advised in the athlete's meeting the night before. The whole thing was so surreal. I lost my balance a few times in my heels through sheer nerves but thankfully no tripping occurred! I felt so confident. Strutting my walk and enjoying the whole experience was what I was relishing in. All I could hear were people screaming my name with every pose that was executed. Anton and I had the best support around us.

Executing the routine not only felt surreal, but even more so an indescribable moment. You only ever really truly understand what it feels like until you do it. I can imagine dancers and actors and actresses probably feel very similar to a performance like this one. But the amount of confidence you have to pretend to have even if you're overcome with nerves is crazy. I felt so overwhelmed with love and support from so many people that day. The number of Instastories I was tagged in, the people that came to support us was more than I had hoped for. I still couldn't believe this was me.

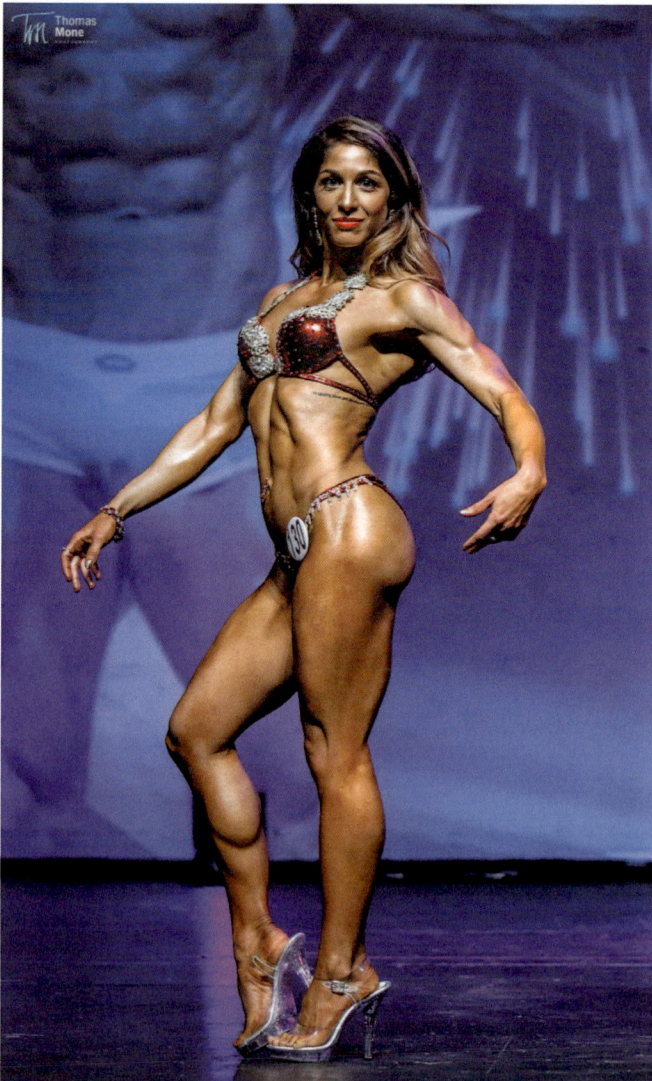

Front pose, hold. Side pose, hold. Back pose, hold. Strut the walk to the right, pose. Strut the walk to the left, pose. Walk to the back and fade into the darkness.

After doing my routine three times for each category, it was like a big weight had been lifted off my shoulders and all I could think about afterwards was the food. At this point there was still so much waiting around. If I were to win a Pro card (certifying you placing 3rd, 2nd or 1st), I would have the opportunity to be called for the Pro show straight after and that was something I would have to think about. All you can really do is snack and wait for the results. I'm pretty sure that night I had consumed a whole packet of rice cakes, some jam and a whole load of grapes! (Grapes are good for the dehydration apparently). I decided not to make any hasty decisions about the Pro show, and maybe decide IF it happened.

As soon as I was called on stage again, the nerves kicked in with a vengeance. Believe it or not, it is so hard to stay posed when you're dehydrated, tired and starving! Of course I knew I was never going to place in Bikini (I had way too much muscle mass for that category) but when it was Miss Wellness all I could hear was people shouting my name and my number: 'Number 130, number 130!'

As soon as a short blonde was called up for 5th place in my heart, I knew I would never place. But when my number was called for 4th place, I just could not believe it. The elevation in that moment was unbelievable. I was shocked but relieved AND so happy that I knew this wasn't all for nothing.

I ran up to collect my trophy and the smiling beam on my face stayed on there for the best part of two weeks. I had also placed 5th in Fitness.

I didn't end up winning a Pro Card, (this defines you from others as part of the elite and means you can follow a genuine career as a professional bodybuilder and are more open to financial opportunities). Being one place away from winning one (you must be 3rd to get it) I still felt a winner, nonetheless. In my head I was a winner because I'd placed in my first show, and I had done something that for a very long time was impossible. My life was going to be different from this moment onwards. It was going to be great.

To be honest, I was more excited to see how Anton would place. Watching him on stage was the proudest moment I ever felt. Knowing that everything I had become and learned was all because of him. That night he became World Champion, winning the whole entire show. I just knew it. I knew he would place but deep down I knew he would be the best, because he was.

He was number one!

As he collected his belt, we packed up our millions of bags and went out to see everyone. Wow, we felt like celebrities! With tired legs, climbing the round staircase to the lobby, voices started to echo louder and louder. As we reached the top, a metaphorical symbol of our successes, excited faces surrounded us. Everyone hugged and screamed, phones were flashing in front of our faces and I'm pretty sure we had an emotional family hug in the car park and to my surprise, even my mum cried.

It was such a turning point in my life. Not just because I had done this, actually placed 5th and 4th in two categories but more because now was the start of my new life. Teaching was behind me, I was no longer the old me and it did make me emotional thinking that in two days' time, I would be starting my PT course, and I was embracing this daunting but exciting new career venture.

L was amazing that night and got Anton and I pizzas (of course I got a veggie stuffed crust) and we ate it ravenously in the car. There is a very funny video of me tucking in, after 6 months of not having anything 'normal' to eat and I just remember my poor manners as I started talking in between chews saying how amazing it tasted. As the doughy texture touched my lips, I was in bliss. The stringy cheese felt heavenly, and I took bite after bite until I couldn't eat anymore. I managed 3 slices of pizza and 2 slices of Chocolate cake. I had never felt so full in my life. But it was so worth it.

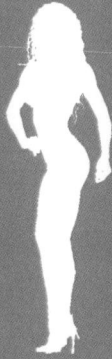

Watching him on stage was the proudest moment I ever felt. Knowing that everything I had become and learned was all because of him.

By the time we got home it was late and I had to be up early in the morning to drive to Wales (or L to drive me to Wales) to do my photoshoot with AK Anakelle. I cannot believe I'm admitting this now, but I slept in my makeup from the show and only topped it up slightly for the shoot-I didn't even shower! I was so hyped from the day it took me ages to get to sleep.

As I laid my tired head on the pillow, little flashbacks of the stage lights, the screams of cheers, the sparkling bikinis enveloped my mind, and I was already buzzing for the next show in two weeks' time.

Upon waking the next morning, I felt like I'd been hit by a bus. The headache was unreal from the dehydration and the tiredness was horrible too. Knowing I was sitting in the car for a gazillion hours too was unnerving knowing in 2 weeks' time I'd be stepping on stage at Pure Elite and would still need to stay on track. I remember having a meltdown in the car because that day My Fitness Pal stopped working (the app I used to log all my foods) and I was having a heart attack!

Looking back now, you realise how abnormal that is for your whole life, your emotions, your entire mood to be controlled by a food app. My body felt tired and overall, it felt like a very bad hangover, all I wanted was to curl on my sofa in my dressing gown and sleep. I may have nodded on and off at times during the journey but eventually after a caffeine hit, I stared out of the window watching grey turning to green. We had arrived in Wales.

Shooting with AK was amazing. The pictures were stunning. I still look at them now and think wow, I could be on the front of a magazine. She made me feel so comfortable and so sexy. I loved every moment. The shoot lasted an hour as she directed me where to look, where to place my hands, when to change outfits.

The very long drive on the way home was even more stressful knowing that I still had to train legs as it was a Monday and the very next day, I would have to be up bright and early to start my course. Anton was telling me not to bother, but I just couldn't imagine it, I remained so focused. When you're in the zone, you're in the zone.

After scrolling on Instagram and seeing he was training legs, I felt so envious I had decided I didn't care how late it would be, I was also going to train before the end of the day. I had never felt so tired, but I still rocked up to the Hertfordshire Golf Club around 8.30 p.m. and got it done. The next day was the start of my new career.

The next four weeks were a crazy blur. Having to pass the course even when prepping again for Pure Elite was tough, especially in peak week where I had exams to pass but my brain wasn't functioning properly. It was great having some advantage in a way over the others in the class in terms of my knowledge and experience. A lot of them were young kids fresh out of college and I admit feeling so out of place amongst them. I couldn't relate to these people. I got the impression that quite a few of them were completing this course out of boredom, or something just to pass the time, or something to keep them ticking over until they decided what they wanted to do with their lives. That wasn't the case for me, I wanted this to be a serious career to excel in. It wasn't that I thought I was better than them, I just felt quite confident because I knew what I wanted. I wasn't in the same stage of their life. This realisation gave me some sort of confidence that although I was out of my comfort zone, I was going to be alright in starting this new job and I couldn't wait to begin.

I admit I didn't enjoy the second show Pure Elite as much as Miami Pro. It wasn't because I didn't place but it was because it felt like more of a rushed day.

My makeup was only finished a second before I was supposed to step on stage and maybe because it was further away in Margate, we only had our mum and stepdad there so the atmosphere felt a bit flat. I won't repeat what it was like but in terms of the waiting around and the feelings on stage, they were all the same. I just remember feeling freezing, more so than ever. Margate is by the sea so the draught coming into the venue was horrible and doors were inconsiderately left open. I sat with my coat on the whole time until I went on stage, wanting it to be over instead of relishing every moment. That night I looked bloated on stage, but I was past caring about food, knowing it was the last show and knowing it was an even longer day. We didn't get out of there until gone 11.00 p.m. and so that night after Anton became World Champion (again) we stayed up until 3.00 a.m. eating pizza! This time I felt incredibly sick and passed out on the bed in a food coma. But it was done. It was over. It was complete.

I was right in taking this leap and willing to prove everyone else wrong, who believed it too much of a risk.

Many people get serious post show blues when it is all over. For weeks I kept saying to Anton how much I wanted to rewind time and relive it all again because of how amazing the experience was. To be honest, I felt genuinely happy for the most part that they were over. I do believe it was probably because I had a new path to be ecstatic about. I was qualified, I was starting a new and exciting job and, in a place, where I once began as a client. The future was not bleak.

Working at B********t felt like home, and it was as if I'd always been there. We had the best team ever. To this day I am still best friends with Charlotte who became one of the only other female PTs there. The relationship we all had was strong; we were all friends as well as colleagues. We'd enjoy our breaks in between clients in the staffroom, go for coffees, take walks and we were all on the same page in terms of our love of training, work ethic, passion, and values.

It was the beginning of a new journey for me and the beginning of many fitness journeys for my future clients. But I was ready to prove to myself I was right in taking this leap and willing to prove everyone else wrong, who believed it too much of a risk.

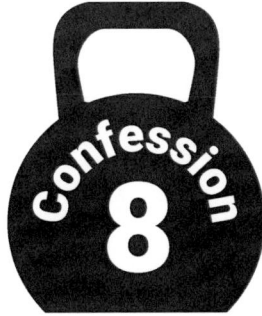

The Day After

*"If you can't control your peanut butter,
you can't expect to control your life."*
Bill Watterson

The day after was a whirlwind and felt very surreal. The last show was in Margate, and I woke up in the Travelodge feeling absolutely shattered from the excitement of the night, not to mention eating pizzas until the early hours and passing out at 3am.

An early riser like me, Anton was in the room next to us and so I messaged him to discuss the events of the previous night. I knocked excitedly on his door.

We sat on his bed, as the sun poured in from the open window, reminiscing the previous night's events. We kept repeating over and over how we couldn't believe this happened, how he had made World Champion *again*. I will never forget his words when I questioned him about how he was feeling knowing he had won the entire show for a second time: 'It doesn't change anything Tash, I'm still going to go into work on Monday, I'm still the same person.' Those words have forever stuck in my head. They sum up and confirm the amazing person that my brother is and how humble he is beyond belief. I really do believe if he won the lottery tomorrow, money wouldn't change him.

About an hour later we went back to my room to wake L up, who was still dead to the world. The plan was to go to Frankie and Benny's for breakfast, before the drive home. Without wasting any more of the day, we quickly dressed, checked our tanned selves out in the mirror and left.

This was the first time we would be eating out together in over six months! It felt so alien to me. What was even more strange is that I couldn't decide what I wanted to eat.

Unfortunately, indecisiveness around food is one of the things you have to work on in recovery after competing. I kept going back and forth, changing my mind, many things going on in my head: I should go for the healthiest option, I should go with what I really wanted. Your mind is forever playing tricks on you with regards to what you want, overanalysing if something is a good or bad decision, whether you've ordered enough food, whether it's too much and in many ways, being restricted to certain foods makes way for demonisation of other foods.

After scanning the menu for what felt like half an hour, the waiter approached. Anton's impatience was made blunt when he remarked 'Just make a decision Tash!' So in the end I went with two poached eggs on a muffin with smoked salmon and hollandaise sauce. There is a video that L took of me the moment I took the first bite. I look like someone eating for the first time, it made me feel so happy in the moment and relieved. This was the closest thing to "normal" I had experienced in six months.

Then it started.

Like an evil spell, it was cast over me. Little did I know what was yet to come in the months to follow and how my relationship with food would never be the same again. Driving back in the car and only having just had breakfast, I couldn't help staring at the snack bags next to me. It was the forbidden fruit. It contained a Salted Caramel cake (big enough for six people), a whole packet of Biscoff biscuits and a whole jar of Biscoff spread.

Like an evil spell, it was cast over me. Little did I know what was yet to come in the months to follow.

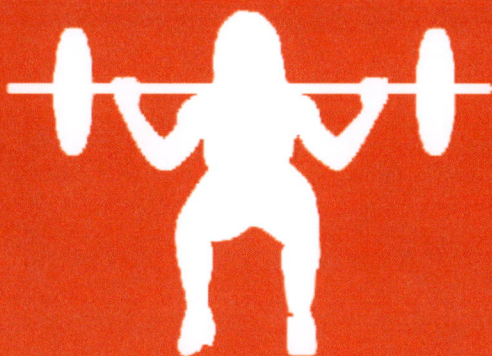

I couldn't help myself; the urge was too strong. I ravenously opened the cake and devoured it in record time. As I continued the drive, I started feeling nervous that other drivers or even L or Anton would see me eating (early signs of shame around eating) so I left the bag on the floor and kept picking from the Biscoff packet, stuffing two and then four biscuits at a time; the speed of each bite getting progressively quicker. This carried on for about twenty minutes and then I started dipping the biscuits in the spread and eating uncontrollably as if they were going to disappear before my eyes. The crumbs were all over my lap, over the floor, over the car seats and I didn't even care.

I looked a state.

All I cared about was consuming these goodies. Some crumbs were moist from falling from my mouth and embedded themselves into the seats, but I just kept going, stains which would linger and be a constant reminder of my binging for months to come. Glancing at my face in the rear-view mirror, beige stains remained on my mouth, wet, sticky crumbs welded around my lips.

Wiping my mouth impulsively with the back of my hand, I thought to myself that I didn't even feel as full as I thought. Little did I know my hunger hormone and satiety hormone were working inefficiently from months of dieting: "Decreased fat mass in an individual triggers the body's homeostatic endocrine response as it is a sign the body is starving. As a result, there is a decreased release of leptin, which is the hormone responsible for fullness and satiety released by adipose tissue. With the decrease in leptin, the anorexigenic hormone, the antagonistic response is the increase in ghrelin, the orixigenic hormone, which stimulates appetite... Many people will shovel thousands of calories within a matter of a few hours after the show... With long periods of dieting, metabolic adaptation occurs which leads to adaptive thermogenesis, increased mitochondrial efficiency, and increased hunger." (Davidson, Mandell, Fagan (Bodybuilders Develop Binge Eating Disorders Post Competition: A Survey- Rutgers University (rutgers-lib-51572_PDF-1.pdf)

Everything had gone. I wasn't me. I let it happen. I then dismissed it ever happened. It felt like I had done something wrong. I'm pretty sure I didn't tell Anton and kept it a secret; a very bad sign, associating food with shame, guilt, and secrecy.

Back at Anton's we continued to reminisce the events of the last twenty-four hours. To end the weekend with a bang, we arranged a celebratory Greek meal out.

L and I got home, and L's brother had arrived to drop our dog Gurgi off after looking after him the whole weekend. All I kept thinking about was the meal out, not an alien habit having food this much on my mind, but certainly a heightened awareness. I was almost wishing his brother to leave so we could go to the restaurant earlier. I was feeling edgy and distracted, finding it incredibly difficult to sit still. The urge and the want growing inside of me, spiralling to the surface.

I will never forget that night, simply because it was the most disgusting I have ever felt in my life. After all the cake and the biscuits and spread, I behaved like a person tasting food for the first time. We went out to a lovely Greek restaurant nearby and I ate *everything*: dips, endless amounts of pitta bread, chicken, salad, and chips and went home to binge for another hour with Anton.

It appears a funny prospect when you try and explain to someone that the binge eating is so bad that you do not sit still for longer than five minutes. The endless steps back and forth to the kitchen whilst opening and closing cupboards and raiding the fridge, probably meant our steps had overshot 12k!

We devoured the baklava that the restaurant gave us to take home and then I even defrosted a chocolate fudge cake that I had made previously (and deliberately frozen) to stop myself from eating it. What was the point of me even doing that?

L was horrified.

At first, he thought it was funny but then explained much later that it was the most uncomfortable thing he had ever witnessed, simply because nothing was more important than food to us. Mid binge, he took a video on his phone which I have never had the guts to post. Despite feeling the worst I've ever felt, my belly was bloated beyond belief, it looked so strange because you could still see my 6 pack. I looked like an alien. I'm pretty sure I went to the toilet quite a few times the next day practically because it was like I'd eaten a year's worth of food in one sitting and my tummy couldn't handle it! My tummy didn't feel normal for about a week. But undeniably, my only comfort was knowing I had gone to bed with a full belly for the first time in half a year.

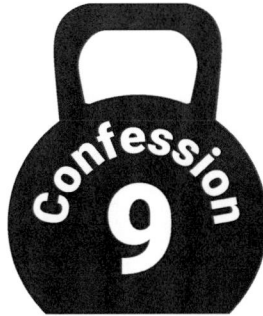

Relationships

" Lots of people want to ride with you in the limo. But you want someone who'll help you catch the bus."
Oprah Winfrey

Before I speak more in the next chapter of my road to recovery, this chapter is one that was vital to be written. Truth: competing changes your relationships forever. Whether it is with a partner, spouse, best friend, mother, the change is inevitable, and in the worst cases, irreparable. Relationships become most strained especially when you are three to four weeks out.

You're tired beyond belief, even talking or laughing is a struggle, you are hangrier (get it? hungrier and angrier= hangrier) Because you are more sensitive and emotional, your patience goes downhill. You are almost killing yourself. It is at this point that although you are in the leanest condition and in most cases the leanest you will ever be in your life; you are at your unhealthiest and unhappiest.

I was lucky that I knew before I even started prep how it would change me. Closer towards show day my entire personality proved just that. I found myself only ever talking about food; whether I was complaining I was hungry, or conjuring a list of all the lovely, sweet treats I would have after show day. My patience wore thin. Anyone close to me or around me would irritate me.

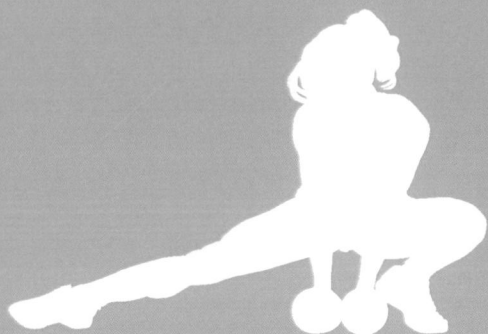

Truth: competing changes your relationships forever.

I became withdrawn.

Many things started annoying me about other people's lives. It could be their relationship, the fact that they had no hobbies, or the fact that they didn't give a shit about their health or just their laziness. It's like this evil judgemental side came out of me, someone I do not recognise, deep down it was not me. I became bold, risking hurting other people's feelings.

I recall an encounter with my mother who I am extremely close to. I told her some home truths about her relationship, and it drove me away from her in many ways. Even my own best friend of eleven years told me after recovery how different I was at the time. I was shorter, blunter and exhibited a lack of empathy.

It was only until after my competition that my best friend confessed, she didn't recognise me during this time. She noticed how drained and different I had become, and only contacted me in the mornings when she rightly ascertained I was at my most energetic and felt most like myself. Those early hours were the only time I still resembled the person she knew.

It's hard because when you are in this zone and so so close to the show, nothing rises above it in its level of importance, nothing and no one. It comes first beyond everything. Competing will always be one of the most selfish sports to embark on. You question when a friend asks you out or asks you to do something that doesn't involve food because you think of your tiredness levels. As terrible as this sounds, I remember the thought that came into my head, worried that a family member would die nearer the time, making me so anxious that I wouldn't be able to compete. The anxiety of failing or not getting to that day after everything I'd invested in, was at its highest.

More annoyingly, because food always came first, everything had to be timed fastidiously. If I was going out, I would need to really think about how long. I'd have all my meals ready and prepped just in case I wasn't back home in time to cook. Spontaneity was thrown out the window. Everything was done in the same way every single day to military precision. In all honesty, it took me a long time to let go. Weighing everything everyday became a norm and trying my best to do anything that stopped me from thinking about food, dreaming about food or coming off track. It's an abnormal life that became my lifestyle.

Nothing rises above it in its level of importance, nothing and no one. It comes first beyond everything.

L would always ask if I was up to doing anything before we committed to any plans with friends. It would never be the question: 'Would you like to go to X's house?' It would be: 'Are you too tired to go to X's house...? We would often go out and I would just watch him eat, I would stick with coffee. We didn't eat out together for months. Anyone knows how this can impact your relationship. Bearing in mind his ex-wife had a severe eating disorder, it certainly triggered a lot of emotions within him, which I just couldn't give my attention to. Although we did our very best, there are only so many outings you can have without involving food.

Our relationship changed. Especially as a woman, your hormones are practically non- existent, and your libido diminishes completely. Of course, this can impact any relationship and can be very hard on a male partner especially: "A study by the University of North Carolina on people's exercise habits and libido levels revealed that excessive exercise can kill desire. It showed that the exhaustion people experience from training leaves some too tired to want anything else but sleep... Extreme exercise can lead to under-functioning pituitary gland, meaning low levels of testosterone and oestrogen." (Magwaza 2017) All your energy is used on training, and you don't have any left, and having sex is the last thing you want to do. As a man, it is hard to accept, every man has physical needs. Your partner doesn't want it anymore, they are forever focused on themselves, on their food, on their training and their shows. It makes them question the relationship, whether their partner is still attracted to them. If L wasn't

L I don't think my relationship would have survived at the time. To be able to do a show, your partner needs to understand something that they've never experienced to support you and I had that endless, relentless support from him.

In my darkest hours, especially when I was most hungry at night, he would remind me how much closer I was to the end. When I was at my wits end as we got into bed he would softly say, 'Just another x number of weeks to go, you can do this.' It also helped that he was into his running, not the sort of person that ate takeaways every night or ate badly; there wasn't that much temptation around me at home.

He would often ask permission to eat in front of me because he could sense how hungry I was. This is so endearing for someone who will never experience what I accomplished. Once he had pizza and didn't even mind that I asked to touch the cheese with my finger, I laugh out loud now when I think about it. Without tasting it, this odd request was the closest I would ever get to this pizza. He accepted other unusual behaviours such as when I sat looking through recipe books or scroll social media looking at recipes or videos of food.

Because L was a vegetarian (eventually turned pescatarian) for a long time, I was used to us eating different foods from the start of our relationship, so it made it all slightly easier. However, I guess the hardest thing for him when I was on prep was that my behaviour was very similar to that of someone with an eating disorder, in terms of my level of control and perfection of eating. This certainly affected his emotional state. Even though being on prep is not an eating disorder, the symptoms and behaviours are very similar: restriction, strict eating windows and avoiding social eating.

Baked oats were my daily breakfast. To explain to you L's level of support, one day I had forgotten that my oats were in the oven, and they burnt to a crisp. I had popped out quickly and received a call from L: 'Tash, I don't want you to panic because I have sorted it, but you left your baked oats in the oven, and they burned. So, I just want you to know that I went on your My Fitness Pal and remade the exact amount for you to the gram'.

I came home, stepped into the kitchen, the freshly baked oat smell filling the flat and hugged him for a very long time, the newly baked oats sitting on a cooling rack on the kitchen counter. That was true love. He knew how much this meant to me and he made it mean a lot to him too.

I have heard that prep has had the capability to end relationships, some left completely irreparable after. I guess that was very brave of L and I to be confident enough that we would still work out, which we did for another three years. To be honest, it never even entered my mind, maybe because we had been through so much in the past and if we had got through that (for those that know our history) then we truly believed we could get through anything.

The relationship with Anton was my only source of stability, because he was on this whirlwind journey with me, always present, the secure anchor amid the challenges and sacrifices. Our shared commitment to this sport deepened our bond but also created a barrier, making us feel like outsiders in our own social circles. We found ourselves only able to be around people who cared about the bodybuilding sport, gravitating towards those who truly understood our lifestyle. These selected few helped us stay motivated yet, at the same time, disconnected us from those who couldn't relate.

Relationships are challenging anyway, even when you're your most consistent self, but as we know, you aren't the *real you*, especially towards the end. While this journey in bodybuilding and my relentless dedication to improving my physique led to significant personal growth and achievement, it also created a permanent distance to those around me, changing the types of relationships I chose to have with others thereafter.

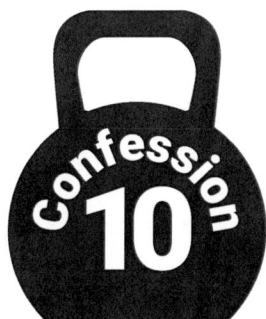

The Road to Recovery

"We can't hate ourselves into a version of ourselves we can love."
Lori Deschene

This is the hardest chapter I will write. I honestly do not even know where to begin. Talking about eating disorders and disordered eating is incredibly hard, especially in the bodybuilding community. The focus on social media is usually on showcasing lean, sculpted bodies, rarely addressing the true, often ugly, struggles behind the scenes, behind those perfect pictures. I'm warning you; this may possibly be the longest chapter in this whole memoir. There are so many aspects to the road to recovery and this is the topic that nearly all bodybuilders *never admit* to themselves and to others. The pressure to maintain a perfect image often overshadows the reality of disordered eating and its impact on mental, emotional and physical health and the evil consequences of getting down to a shredded physique from the many months of dieting. Only the individual that goes through this has it contained like a Pandora's box in their mind. Although I have written Instagram posts here and there about the disordered and binge eating, I am writing everything now to every minute detail as best as I can. Sharing this truth is daunting but so necessary to bring awareness to an often hidden and taboo issue.

I want to be remembered for being that individual in the fitness industry who revealed the truth about this side (the dark side) to competing. And here are my true confessions and experiences about this subject.

As someone who has suffered much of my life with Binge Eating Disorder (B.E.D.), I find that many use the term too loosely in everyday life: 'I binged so much on chocolate on Saturday night' or 'I binged so much I nearly ate a whole packet of biscuits.' If only this is as far as B.E.D. takes you. I can tell you now, it rules your life so much, there is no line, there is no stop at one packet of biscuits. The reality is, most people cannot comprehend not drawing the line at one packet of biscuits, or even two, or reaching the point of actually throwing up, or even the point where you are trying so hard to stick your toothbrush to the back of your throat to erase the shame you felt with everything you've eaten—yes, this has happened to me too.

The following report *The Binge and the Brain* sums it up perfectly: "Genuine binge eating is recurrent and debilitating—physically and emotionally... Loss of control is what distinguishes a binge from simple overeating... being unable to stop consuming food despite a strong desire to stop, a feeling of fullness, eating alone because of being embarrassed about how much one is eating, or even a sense that the food's taste is no longer appealing. Some also report eating much more rapidly than normal... In severe binges, the drive for overindulgence may cause patients to consume raw pancake mix, entire loaves of bread... however lacking in taste they may be. The patient often plans secret eating in advance and carries it out late in the day—and typically experiences disgust, depression, and guilt afterwards." (Ely and Cusack 2015)

Many people suffer with it more than you realise, whether bodybuilding or not. What's worse is that you can walk past an average-looking person in the street, not necessarily overweight or underweight, and only if you spent enough time with them daily or participated in discussions with them about food, may you come to realise that it is a disorder that can be very easily hidden. If only you could see into the mind of these normal-looking people who internally, grapple with deep emotional pain, anxiety or depression, all because of food.

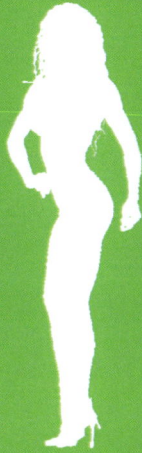

I want to be remembered for being that individual in the fitness industry who revealed the truth.

"Currently, about sixty percent of diagnosed cases are in women... Indeed, research into the neural mechanisms of BED is still in its infancy, so there is no specific treatment for the disorder." (Ely and Cusack 2015) This is what makes this disorder probably the loneliest place to be; there is no way out because there is no real help for it unlike anorexia whereby you can be hospitalised, or it's visibly obvious that the person suffers. The cycle of overeating and guilt creates an isolating prison, but with no actual guard keeping you there except your own mind. You're in control of what you put into your mouth but you're not. Embarrassment makes it harder to seek support or understanding from others *especially* in the bodybuilding world, making the disorder seem insurmountable.

Before I go into my Binge Eating Disorder (B.E.D.) after shows, something quite common for many competitors, even for those who have never suffered with this disorder before, it's important to understand my history and relationship with food a bit more. If I were to psychoanalyse myself, it's fair to say dieting has always been traumatic. When I've lost drastic weight in the past, it has been due to stress (in my early years as a teacher in particular). You may also recall in an earlier chapter where binge eating wasn't something I wasn't unfamiliar with as Head of English. Seeking comfort in food to escape the stresses of my job and relationship, meant dieting and dropping weight always had negative associations in adulthood. Even post show, the trauma of dealing with the mental side of eating, affected my confidence and body image was a P.T.S.D. in itself.

Let's rewind time. The earliest memory I have of secret eating was when I was about six years old. It was always a rule that me and my brother never took anything from the kitchen unless we asked our parents, that was made very clear. We had to ask permission to take food from the fridge if we were hungry, and sometimes if it was too close to dinner the answer would be: "No, you'll spoil your dinner."

I remember this episode as clear as day. My dad worked in the city as a manager of a Cleaning Company called OCS which I believe doesn't exist anymore, and meant he left the house at 4am, but always finished by the afternoon. Therefore, he would be home to look after us after school until my mum got home later from work. Anton was probably sleeping at the time, but I remember planning out this secret eating episode.

CITV was on in the background and habitually my dad would fall asleep, snoring loudly with his foot crossed over the other against the dark, mahogany coffee table. I didn't want to ask permission to eat, so I waited until he fell into that deep slumber and tiptoed quietly into the kitchen, turning back a few times to check he hadn't woken.

Phew, I made it to the kitchen.

48 King's Road, in Edmonton was a typical 80s style house. Everything in the kitchen was brown. Cream wallpaper with fruit bowl emblems across it, the window overlooking the conservatory decorated with ugly curtains that my mum had made herself from her sewing machine. I guess before the birth of the internet, people had time to do such mundane tasks.

Crossing the cold, hard floor, I stared at the cupboard straight ahead of me, where the biscuit tin was kept, on the highest shelf imaginable so Anton and I didn't have easy access. Again, holding my breath and looking over my shoulder for the last time, I jumped up onto the kitchen counter, freezing at the same time as balancing on my toes and holding my breath again for any signs of my dad walking in.

Feeling so pleased with myself, I opened the cupboard door in slow motion and stared at the biscuit tin before me. For those of you that remember those typical 90s biscuit tins, they were difficult to open. This tin was also cream coloured but with an extensively stiff aluminium lid that made the loudest racket every time it was opened.

I held my breath again.

My fingertips caressed the lid, and I felt the greatest satisfaction imagining what the next few minutes would feel like when my lips touched the edge of the first biscuit. Attempting to avoid any loud noise, with all my strength amidst a bit of a struggle, I opened it with great force, tucking the tin under my right armpit because I thought it would camouflage the noise.

It opened.

The smell of the sweet sugars hit me. The biscuits were either the NICE biscuits or the malty milks; the ones with the cow picture on, I cannot remember exactly. But I had succeeded. Over the course of the next few minutes, I practised eating in silence and in great haste, eating a few biscuits and then staring down into the bottom of the tin, ensuring to stop so it didn't look like too many had disappeared.

Feeling satisfied I rearranged the remaining biscuits, so they looked more spread out (forgive my child-like mind) and carefully closed the cupboard, jumping down and landing so lightly on my feet I was impressed with myself.

Walking boldly back into the living room, I ensured to wipe my mouth with the back of my sleeve in case any crumbs remained and lay on the sofa watching the next programme credits light up the TV screen, listening to the audible lamentations of my dad's snores.

So there you have it, my earliest memory of secret eating.

If we fast forward time to a couple of years later when I was eight or nine years old, it is vital to understand where my negative views of dieting came from.

My mum was *always* on a diet. Married with this she would always insult herself with comments such as 'Eugh, I'm so fat... I feel so fat... I've put on weight... I need to lose weight.' Or, 'I've eaten too much, I feel sick.' Call it damaging and these are the only comments I ever remember, and they are all negative. As far as I can remember, she has never had a positive body image. From a young age, I would attend Weight Watchers meetings with her, eat her Weight Watchers sweets and just observe her eating. I even remember asking her if I could write down my "points" in a Weight Watchers diary like her and so instead of telling me no, that I didn't need to worry about calories, she got me a diary and encouraged me.

I became exposed to this idea of dropping weight, tracking food and tracking points. My understanding of dieting was wholly consumed by the guilt and shame of overeating by my mother and her negative body image and self-esteem.

Fast forward a few years later. Tash, eleven years old.

Every weekend my *yiayia* (grandma in Greek) would come over. She was by that time diagnosed with Lewey's Body Disease (a form of Motor Neurone Disease) which meant she would be very slow. It is a progressive illness whereby your muscles gradually die, and all movement is eliminated. Sadly, she is no longer with us but she was bedridden for the last twenty years of her life, unable to eat, move or talk. "Motor neurone disease is a rare condition that progressively damages parts of the nervous system. This leads to muscle weakness… also known as amyotrophic lateral sclerosis (ALS), occurs when specialist nerve cells in the brain and spinal cord called motor neurones stop working properly. This is known as neurodegeneration." (nhsinform)

Motor Neurone Disease is probably one of the most insufferable diseases out there, simply because you are not dying, you are merely fading away, as every liberation is taken away from you. From walking, to hugging, to touching, to talking. You become a vegetable. On this particular Saturday, it was dinner time and Mum was calling Anton and I to come and sit at the table.

It took one comment. That comment has stayed with me my whole life.

My *yiayia* who it's fair to say was never the tactful type, said to me, 'Natasha Mou, you've got too much on your plate, you'll get fat.' That's all it took. I'd barely even tucked in, yet for the remainder of the meal

I sat with my head down, hands clasped staring at the peas on my plate, counting them one by one and fighting back tears.

How I didn't develop an eating disorder after this was astonishing, yet it's safe to say when I look back, every year that passes I have little epiphany moments or memories that somehow surface and make me realise why I am the way I am.

Comments such as these are hurtful and should *never* be made to young children.

There were other occasions where my *yiayia* would openly say to my mum in front of my dad, Anton and I: 'Miranda, you've put on weight' or 'Miranda you've got fat.' At the time, I was too young to understand how much my *yiayia* belittled my mum, making her feel worthless. I do believe my mum's issues somehow are deep rooted with treatment such as this from her own Mother.

Only recently, when the subject of my *yiayia* has come up, has my mum opened up to me about her issues with food. She recalls that my *yiayia* would give her "the stare." My mum explained how she would get anxiety walking across the living room when she was in her teenage years because my *yiayia* would give her this piercing stare, eyeing her up at the same time as saying 'Miranda, I think we've put on a little bit of weight.' Adults claim that children are not perceptive, but the fact that my mum still remembers such trauma at the age of sixty, is proof: "Research linking specific parental behaviours (i.e., emphasis on appearance, commentary about body size and appearance) with body image dissatisfaction... suggests that a family culture that emphasises appearance and thinness might be associated with both increased disordered eating and body image dissatisfaction." (Kluck 2010)

My parents have been divorced for over fifteen years, but my mum even told me how when she had her wedding dress fitting, her mother took complete control and advised the fitter to avoid adding ruffles and bows in order my Mum could "look slimmer". These behaviours and comments are gut wrenching, yet they were normalised because they were said so frequently. I am only thankful that my mum has NEVER insulted my weight. She has only ever made me feel confident and complimented me, whatever my size. So, thank you Mum for the confidence you have always instilled in me, you've only ever made me feel good about myself, always.

Tears sting my eyes and I'm wracked with guilt as I write this because there have been times when at family gatherings, we have poked fun at my mum's weight, to which she has also poked fun at herself. Usually, she's instigated it, whether it be a picture someone has taken and shocked looking at herself and exclaim, 'Eugh is that really me?!' It is only now years later that I see how damaging that is. I regret it so much. And Mum, if you're reading this, I am truly sorry. I wish I could rewind time. Just a word of warning to you; before you comment on someone's weight, think very carefully about your choice of words.

Fast forward again to 2019, Natasha Kostalas, Competitor Number 130.

After show day, after you have the biggest ego boost because the comments by others are: 'I want to look like you', 'you look amazing,' I want your back and 6 pack'.

What then?

What happens when time goes by, people forget you ever competed, you pile on the pounds, you don't even realise how bad your body has become in terms of hormonal function, normal bodily functions and most importantly eating and hunger levels, not to mention your confidence and self-esteem which completely disintegrates. What does that make you when that time has passed? Who are you, *really*? I don't think you even know: "... the most psychologically devastating aspect that fuels the post-contest depression is the loss of lean condition." (Harris, 2020) "One factor is a quick drop in neurotransmitters. I'm sure you've all heard about the uplifting effects of dopamine and serotonin... To quote an article on tnation.com, dopamine is intensely triggered by the competitive mindset... When you enter that zone, dopamine is released in heaps. So basically, when the competition is over, you don't have the same number of happy drugs circulating in your system, so that leads to a more depressed state... So just from a chemical standpoint, it makes sense why there can be such a feeling of change." (Harris, getpoised.net)

My last show was November 2019. Being so close to Christmas you could say that in a way it is the worst time to come out of a show because you are surrounded by food. It is the festive season and there are so many family functions to attend (all pre-Covid of course). You could say my biggest mistake was eating what I wanted and not being able to stick to a proper reverse diet: "Reverse dieting is a post-diet eating strategy that slowly increases your calorie intake (over weeks or months) to prevent weight gain as you return to your previous calorie levels. It has been popular in the bodybuilding community as a way to prevent rapid weight gain after a competition." (Bourgeois 2024) To be fair to Anton as my Coach, he did strongly advise me of how to do this, but I just couldn't fight the temptation. To be honest, I do believe I would have experienced the same things, with the same results and consequences even if it wasn't Christmas, so I cannot even use that as an excuse.

As happy as I was with my training regime, I still made mistakes there too. Remember, training was why I wanted to compete in the first place. The strength, the energy, revelling in all of that. But the second biggest mistake I made was thinking that I was still just as strong as I was before I began.

Although I accepted that the weights I was lifting had decreased drastically because I'd gotten weaker, naively I thought I would just bounce back just because I was eating more and I was heavier. This time post show, training changed for the worst. Where I truly believed that I would quickly build my strength back up, I ended up getting injured to the extent that I couldn't really do much.

I kept training normally but noticed that my hip started to hurt during certain exercises, and I would start to feel it doing other day to day activities like walking the dog or getting in and out of my car.

My right shoulder started giving me issues as well. I just kept thinking that I was starting to fall apart. I'm pretty sure I didn't listen well enough when Anton kept saying to me, 'Don't go ham, you don't want to get injured.' Little Miss Invincible Me just thought I'd be fine just because I was eating more food and put on weight.

I want to slap myself for being so overconfident. I rushed the process. My body just couldn't keep up. I was having more fun because I was pushing my strength too quickly. You could say I felt like Superman or Superwoman after taking an antidote for kryptonite. Charlotte, my best friend at the gym I was working at and I were having so much fun training together and I loved training with Anton and the other trainers in our gaps between clients, especially our regular Saturdays at midday when everyone had finished work. It really felt like home.

One Saturday training session, I glanced over at Anton training with two of the other male trainers and I could see them all goading each other in a competition to see who could do the most 20kg press-ups to failure. Of course, I had to join in and there was a video that Anton took which I had to post; the shock and horror on their faces where I had managed to do about twenty or twenty-one reps with a 20kg on my back. It was the most confident I had felt post show.

Both injuries were starting to become so much more painful after this episode. I had to see a physio; in fact, I saw two. They had told me I had a slight hip tear probably from an overload on a hip thrust even though I was still managing 150kg hip thrusts and in addition a rotator cuff again, probably from an overload on a bench press. So, to then be told I couldn't do any bench pressing either barbell or Dumbbell was tough. My hip tear was affecting so many exercises I couldn't do barbell squats, walking lunges, squats, step-ups, split squats, practically no lower body at all. All this lasted six months! I still trained but had to work around all these injuries. It made me realise the damage I had done to my body because of my ego. Despite me feeling down about my training and learning to live with the pain and annoyance of these injuries, I didn't let it stop me from achieving any PBs. To be fair to myself, by 2020 I hit the best PBs I'd ever done in my training career at that time: 105kg squat and 155kg deadlift. My bench press PB wasn't until 2021 (60kg).

The only way in which I felt confident besides the injuries was due to the fact I was starting to really enjoy my training with aiming towards these PBs, but my confidence in terms of my body image was at its all-time low. On the 19th December about six or so weeks post show when my weight had shot up drastically, I decided I needed to post a current physique picture. There were three images, one of me in leggings and sports bra in the gym, at home and another where I was in a sports bra and underwear. I wasn't wearing any makeup either and frankly it was the first time I could bring myself to post on social media in this way. I felt huge although looking at the pictures now, I wasn't. This is what I posted:

I don't want to be that person that only posts "ripped" or super lean pictures of themselves on social media.

Above is my current body composition (no makeup/ no filter. TRUTH: the 'glamour' of comp meant it has taken 1 month and 10 days to have the confidence to post this, as I gradually get used to having more body fat again. TRUTH:

1. *People expect you to look super lean all year round-even comments of surprise when you're seen eating "normal" foods*

2. *You still have "prep habits" For example, making sure your plate is completely clean and you've eaten every last crumb.*

3. *Strength has improved. Current stats: back squats 80kg, front squats 70kg, deadlifts 110kg, hip thrusts 160kg, bench press 45kg it really is strength vs aesthetics*

4. *Injury: eating more, being heavier but lifting heavier has meant I have now developed a shoulder/hip flexor injury. Eating foods with low nutritional value has increased inflammation and not helped this.*

5. *Achieving consistency is still a slow process for me (people can't understand why you can't just be in a deficit again)*

6. *Hormones are still not back to normal, people forget that stage weight was not healthy.*

7. *This is more a psychological process than a physical. It is true when I was told you never look at food in the same way: You overanalyse everything about food- what you're eating, how you're eating it and your own behaviours!*

8. *You do miss the ripped abs and fitting into tiny clothes (I went down to size 6 and even fitted into an aged 11-12 top) but IT IS NOT HEALTHY OR NORMAL*

9. *I am embracing being bigger, will embrace this year long muscle building phase and I have all my performance goals in mind. Was it all worth it to compete? Without a doubt it has been my favourite memory of 2019. Will I compete again? Fingers crossed 2021.*

10. *I want to keep it real and remind people that I am an average person (despite the "glamour" of a show and yes, sometimes you do feel like a catfish!) Training and nutrition really can change your body whether it's being super lean or having higher body fat but you must be confident no matter what.*

11. *Most importantly I will enjoy this part of the process and feel confidence in this skin*

Clearly, I was making excuses for myself for failing my reverse diet.

Number 2 was inspired by someone in the gym (one of the trainers) hurting my feelings. The truth is, this person didn't mean it in a malicious way but because my confidence was incredibly low, I couldn't handle jokes if it was anything to do with my eating habits or my body.

Sitting in the staffroom one day and finishing a yoghurt, this trainer walked in.

Intimidating at times with his serious face, jet black eyes and short cut hair, he was the ultimate alpha male. Trust me, you would never want to get on the wrong side of this guy. Incredibly knowledgeable and an expert in the field of bodybuilding, he was that individual that you would respect immediately, even if that respect was organically from fear. His manner was at times abrupt, yet he was the leader of the pack, a complete alpha, the king of the jungle.

I was so hurt after this episode, merely because he had competed on many occasions yet showed no empathy for the aftermath. His eyes met mine as he observed me trying to spoon out every bit of yoghurt from the pot; 'Not sure you can get any more out of that yoghurt Tash'. The whole room erupted with laughter, yet Anton's face remained quite stern. He understood.

I laughed it off but deep down inside I was so hurt. I was humiliated. I wasn't coping at all with my relationship with food. I was struggling but I was too ashamed to admit it, even to Anton.

For a long period of time, I felt a fraud. I was the victim of Imposter Syndrome-I felt unworthy. I deeply missed all the comments about my abs, about my physique and I felt like a nobody now, now with the hype gone. After that comment, I drove home, uncontrollable tears streaming down my face, mourning what I had been. Clearly, these post-show blues were real, and I was experiencing them. After months of intense preparation and excitement, it was very tough to adjust back into normal, everyday life.

My eating was bad. I daresay, not as bad as other stories I've heard, but still bad. I kept wondering why on earth I couldn't follow macros for one day, bearing in mind I had done so for half a year and to such a meticulous degree. I failed to last one day! I also noticed I was never full (now I know the reasons were due to the inefficiency of the hunger hormones). I would have a 700-calorie meal and I wasn't satisfied. It is such a horrible yet strange feeling because nearly every time I ate, I felt I could keep going until I could burst. I *yearned* to feel full.

I want to talk to you about the cake incident.

After my second show I still had two weeks to complete my PT course. Of course, not really caring enough or seeing the importance of a proper reverse diet, my cravings and hunger levels were through the roof.

One day on a lunch break on the course, I did the unthinkable. I drove to a Marks and Spencer Food Hall and bought a whole Rainbow Birthday Cake. I'm sure you can guess what happens next. Feeling so ashamed and embarrassed to even be seen eating in front of others I sat in my car and nearly devoured the whole thing.

For a long period of time, I felt a fraud. I was the victim of Imposter Syndrome - I felt unworthy.

I felt disgraceful.

I just couldn't stop.

For the people who use the word "binge" too lightly, I'm not sure you really know what a binge is until you have experienced this. I kept going, even using my hands to stuff the sweet, spongy mixture into my mouth, it was as if there was a ticking time bomb and I had to devour it in record time. Before I knew it, my car seats and floor were filling with snowflake-like crumbs.

Even when I started to feel that it was not tasting as nice as at the start, I kept going, it was like I had lost all sense of control. The worst part about it, I was doing it in secret, and I knew deep down how wrong this was. It wasn't even the first time. I felt sick, bloated and disgusting, even more so deeply ashamed. I didn't even have the guts to tell *anyone* about this incident until years later.

I walked sluggishly back into my PT class trying not to think about what I had done. I felt awful in myself as well as a hypocrite. Leaving to go home at the end of the day I remember looking into the black bag, taking a few more handfuls and then stopping. Everything about this incident was dreadful: the binge eating, the effects on my body physically and mentally and the secrecy. You could say I was embarrassed at times to eat in front of people for fear of judgement.

On another occasion, I drove to a petrol station because the urge took over again, swiping some cookies and cake off the shelf and felt so embarrassed to be in the queue purchasing them, because I thought people were looking at me. I felt a tsunami of paranoia wash over me, my eyes bouncing in every direction, my mind racing with the thoughts of scrutiny, convinced everyone was silently critiquing my every move, my self-consciousness and discomfort amplified.

This is the one problem with becoming stage lean, your body just cannot help the aftereffects. Plus, the amount of time it takes to get back to "normal" makes you question what "normal" is anymore. You are never truly content with your body.

One of the most mindfucking things is that you go from being so spot on with calculating macros for such a long period of time, to then feeling like a complete failure when you are unable to track for one day. It makes you think that there is something wrong with you, that you've gone from that extreme to not even lasting a full day with a good eating structure. At one point I questioned whether I needed therapy for this.

Christmas came around and I was indulging in whatever I wanted. I was baking so much to make up for the six months of not being able to do so. Protein cookies, flapjacks, cakes, the lot. I was noticing the softness that was ensuing around my belly and arms and yet I kept going. In the early days when I still had a six pack I was checking constantly to see if it was still there, it became obsessive. I would feel a sigh of relief when it would stare back at me in my reflection but as the weeks and months wore on, its disappearance made me lose my sense of self-worth and confidence, burying me deep into this grave. I ended up avoiding mirrors for a long period of time after that.

Christmas came and went, and L and I travelled to Bruges for the New Year. Anyone who has been to Bruges knows how temptation is EVERYWHERE. Chocolate shops on every corner, bakeries and inviting lavish restaurants. One thing I was very shocked about in Bruges, as lovely as it was, was that the only side you could order was chips. I struggled because every restaurant we went to did not serve vegetables and I was craving them so much. Not to mention the service is slower than any country I've been to. So, when I was hungry, my impatience would erupt.

In the five or so days we were there I would have oats and whey, with a Grenade protein bar and then another bar if we were out for the day. However, my eating behaviours were both contradictory and erratic. Some days I'd skip lunch and the dinners we opted for most of the trip were not of the traditional cuisine. We had American one night (burger and loaded fries) a couple of other nights we tried their cuisine, but I couldn't get any form of chicken that wasn't in pastry, battered or not in a rich creamy sauce. It's fair to say my stomach couldn't handle the trip—I was on the toilet two or three times a day!

During the day we went to the Chocolate Museum and of course I got my mitts on every free sample possible. My greed was reflective of the fact that my hunger hormones were still not working efficiently. I was becoming sick and tired of not feeling full. The level of obsession continued, and I was still obsessively weighing myself every morning. The fact that I packed my weighing scales says it all. I refused to let go of these habits.

Walking around the city I bought a variety of chocolate and even some chocolate spread and some Belgian waffles in a packet. L was horrified that the chocolate spread had gone within twenty-four hours as I sat eating it with the waffles in the hotel room of an evening and grazing on the chocolate, was surprising enough.

On New Year's Eve we were starting to get fed up of the same cuisine so we booked a lovely Thai restaurant. It was the only place we went to that had vegetables! I was craving them so much and this remained my favourite meal of the whole trip. It's strange how even now, not having vegetables for one day is something so out of the ordinary for me.

Of course, I still trained, and we ended up in a great gym just a twenty-five-minute walk from the main city called Gymms Gym and I had my first leg day of 2020 on 2nd January. Training was always something I knew I could never live without, even if I was on holiday and it remained the only consistent thing that made me feel confident.

The Christmas break came and went, and I continued to love my new job, and hands down my love for it has continued to bloom up to this day.

I still get asked the question on occasion whether I miss teaching and I always give the same flat out "no" with a beaming smile. I don't miss the stress, the lifestyle, the marking. At most I miss the kids but having done Kids' training I still have that treasure of working with youngsters. I love the clients, I loved working with my best friends everyday- with Charlotte, Anton, Mike and all the others. I enjoyed my training despite the injuries and my deadlifts were really picking up.

My clients were doing great. I had some great people. One older woman in particular was sixty-seven years old and having never done weight training before lost over 25lbs in less than five months. Another woman who was very small and slight came to me and over her four months she put on over 7lbs and got super strong. Even the other trainers would comment how defined her upper body had become. It was such a privilege having a muscle/ strength building female as they are quite hard to come by; most women want fat loss today. I was getting the hang of the job and was starting to feel confident because the clients were doing well, and I was in an environment I knew so well, as the coach instead of the client.

More clients started in January, and everyone knows that January is the busiest month for everyone in the fitness industry. L, Anton and I had booked New York for April, so we were so excited for that holiday. Life really was great. Almost too great, that often I would feel a sense of paranoia and would anticipate something bad to happen. But I no longer had those horrible Sunday blues that I used to get in teaching, which would usually start at 3.00 p.m.. I loved waking up in the morning, I was happy, I loved everyone around me, and I had never felt so content. Things seemed almost too good to be true.

Every week I was learning. Yes, I didn't feel confident in my body due to the disordered eating and piling on 35lbs, but people knew me, I had that good reputation, and I had my PT to focus on. I learnt even more about perfecting exercises in my own training. I started to grasp coaching, not just counting someone's reps, but really learning more about an individual's mobility and biomechanics. Common injuries would mean I knew how to alter exercises especially having experienced injuries myself. I felt so confident in what I was doing and in terms of sharing my knowledge with others and I could see that the satisfaction I was getting was very similar to what I first felt in teaching, if not stronger.

I was still suffering with amenorrhea and during this time was researching, reading, and listening to podcasts religiously about all the ways I could get my period back. For the first time in my life, *I wanted it back*. I knew it was important for my body and for my hormones to return to working efficiently.

This was the first post where I spoke about it openly:

Amenorrhea

..

This is what many female athletes suffer (myself included since June 2019!)
..

Definition: the absence of a cycle due to dietary changes and reaching very low body fat-basically the red flag (excuse the pun!) that the female body isn't functioning to its full potential. ..

My research on the topic of recovery is to (apparently!):

1. *Increase calories-one nutritionist mentioned eating between 2000-2500 daily*

2. *Put on weight-this definitely happened naturally post show!*
3. *Eating higher fats, for example, salmon/eggs obviously would mean lowering my carbs*
4. *Relieving stress-ensuring I'm getting enough sleep and definitely napping when I feel the need*
5. *One podcast I listened to recently mentioned tapering down the training. I love lifting heavy and not sure how I'm feeling about this one.*
6. *Going back on the pill-DEFINITELY NOT doing this one*
7. *Consistency: in calories/weight maintenance*
..

If you are a female who has or is suffering with this, any suggestions below would be interesting to know! #waitinggame

Some women let years go by without having one, but I knew I was willing to do anything to win it back. I ended up tapering down the training in the end just to relieve the stress my body had been under for so long.

Then, suddenly one day it happened, and I couldn't help but share my good news with my followers:

After 9 months of waiting (I realise I could have had a baby in this time LOL) the day finally arrived.
..

Men, this won't mean anything to you, but ladies, after reading my previous post on suffering with Amenorrhea, I can't express enough the happiness I felt today knowing my body is FINALLY BACK TO NORMAL, post show.
..

Women currently still suffering with Amenorrhea of all kinds whether due to an eating disorder, stress or due to being an athlete, DON'T IGNORE IT. Your body is telling you that your body is not functioning normally.
..

What I've been doing the last 4 months: ..

- *Eating to satiation: yes I'm more consistent than ever following macros but if there were days where I felt more hungry I would eat. I was ranging between 2000-2500 calories over a period of time. I'm currently eating between 1800-2000. It has taken a LONG time to get to a point like now where I can eat a 500cal meal and feel full.*

- *Body fat% increase: I didn't care about my aesthetics, my priority was getting my cycle back. Yes I'm softer but I feel the most normal I've ever felt since competing. • Listening to my body and my hunger. I stopped worrying about how much weight I was gaining and ate- NOT to a point where I felt sick/ bloated, but when I felt satiated. A Science article I read said: "Both estrogen and progesterone influence your appetite, how much you eat, and the regulation and distribution of fat cells. Estrogen -- particularly estradiol, the major component of the estrogen hormone groups -- seems to decrease hunger by directly affecting the brain's appetite center in the hypothalamus". • Tapering down HEAVY HEAVY lifting: I have calmed it down a tad. For example, instead of regular deadlifts and hitting PBs, my coach incorporated dead stops which required me to go lighter.*

- *Sleep and rest: 7-8 hours daily. If I feel super tired I will nap and not feel bad about it.*

- *Being patient: when it's been gone a long time at first you think it's great and I know a lot of you women told me you wish you never got your cycle. But, when it's gone, you don't feel yourself, nothing is functioning in the right way and you don't feel like a woman. #thewaitingameisover #imawomanagain*

The day the miracle happened, I walked proudly into the gym, announcing it to Anton and one of my female clients at the same time. We both started hugging and jumping around the gym. It was unbelievable celebrating my womanhood. Life couldn't get much better (as uncomfortable as I felt in my skin) but I knew my priorities had certainly changed. Training was good, overeating was still an occurrence, but I knew that I would be competing again in 2021. I couldn't keep away from it for too long.

Early March I posted a picture from my photoshoot with Simon Howard:

10 reasons why I will compete again in 2021

Reason 1: the journey and a sense of purpose: it's the slowest process when you're on a 6 month cut and requires A LOT of patience, but I enjoy every day knowing I'm getting a little closer towards that end goal
..

Reason 2: I love how gradually my body transforms, due to science and the manipulation of macros and of course from training which I love over anything else!
..

Reason 3: the buzz on stage: unless you've competed before or you are a regular performer on stage you will know what I mean by this
..

Reason 4: the day: the anticipation and excitement leading up to it; the tan, the bikini, the hair, the makeup and those nail biting minutes before you get on stage
..

Reason 5: how much you come to value food- you take that for granted in the normal everyday when it's always there
..

Reason 6: meeting new people on the day and sharing your journey in conversations, wishing each other luck and knowing you're all in the same boat
..

Reason 7: the confidence it gives you. I've said this before but when you've done it, you honestly feel like anything is possible
..

Reason 8: to prove to myself I can!
..

Reason 9: having the support of family and friends really makes you feel special; their compliments and commendations keep you going, reminding you that even in your darkest (hungrier!) moments it is all worth it!

..

Reason 10: in 2021 I want to be able to see the progress I've made in my body composition compared to the first shows. I will feel like a winner, even if I don't manage to place again

..

Thank you @snhfoto for wonderful photography

I had a direction. Being uncomfortable in my current body was temporary and 4 months after the first shows I was craving those feelings again. The goal was to build as much strength as I could, focusing on hitting those big numbers which I achieved. The end of 2021 seemed far yet it didn't; timing is everything when it comes to competing. I was so happy, so grateful so humble, so privileged to be in the position I was in, it really did feel too good to be true.

One day, I had one of my older female clients (I think this was around January or February 2020) and during a rest period she turned to me with a serious expression on her face and said, 'Have you heard what's happening in China?'

I replied 'no' with a confused expression on my face. What was she talking about?

She seemed so shocked that I was completely unaware. 'It's all over the news and on the radio, I'm surprised you haven't heard.' I didn't want to emphasise that I deliberately avoided watching the news because I was always sick of the negativity and no news is ever good news. She then went on to explain to me that some virus called Corona was spreading and how she was considering cancelling her holiday to Thailand. Admittedly, at the time, not knowing what I know now, I thought it quite extreme. I was shocked and in my head was thinking, well whatever happens I'm still going to New York in April, nothing was going to stop me.

The more conversations I was having in the gym this Corona Virus topic kept circulating and to my surprise, that female client stopped coming to the gym. Again, at the time I thought it quite extreme.

A few days later, a couple of PTs were starting to fall ill with flu-like symptoms and more cancellations ensued.

Another couple of clients stopped coming to the gym and thoughts of how ridiculous this was, encircled my head. I remember thinking, well it's not spread to here so why is everyone getting their back up? Jokes were being made in the staffroom whenever anyone coughed or sneezed and we would all laugh and joke and say, 'Uh oh, Corona!' This was the attitude that everyone had at the time.

Then, it was starting to come on the news that flights to different countries were being cancelled, holidays were being cancelled by airlines. Clients were asking me 'Are you and Anton still going to NY in April?' My response would always be the same, 'Of course! Nothing is going to stop me!' In silence, I would take a big gulp and think, oh gosh, I really hope this stupid virus is not going to ruin the one trip that I have waited my whole lifetime for.

One day I woke up (towards the end of March) and I felt funny. I just didn't feel right *at all*. That's the only way I can describe it. I had a bad headache, and I was definitely beyond my normal level of tiredness. After work on Monday, my usual routine would be to come back home for a few hours, train and then drive back to work for the graveyard shift (6.00 p.m. to 9.00 p.m.).

I got home but the fatigue was vehement, causing me to roll straight into bed. This was certainly not me.

My head was pounding beyond belief that it only felt it was subsiding if I lay down. I thought well, if I have a nap then I could always train afterwards and I'm sure I will feel a little bit better. I set my alarm and when it went off it felt like it could have been 5.00 a.m. I felt like a zombie. But I did what I've always done. I sucked it up and got through the session. I felt much better afterwards. Then the next day it hit me like a tonne of bricks.

In the days following, I felt terrible. Hand on heart I didn't believe for one second that it was Covid, I just thought that it was just a regular cold or flu. Every conversation in the gym was about Covid and then word was getting round that the UK would be in a lockdown. We all laughed it off. I thought to myself what does lockdown actually mean?

Wait, gyms?!

It suddenly struck me that there could be a possibility that I may not be earning money, that I may not be able to train. Then we all thought, no, England is not like other countries. It would never happen! We were burying our heads in the sand.

We carried on business as usual that week, but I felt worse. Another trainer was complaining she was sweating for no reason even though it was still quite cold out and was asking for cover. I was feeling rotten but didn't let on to anyone else. Then Anton also said he was feeling rough. We had no idea. But then it was all over the news that from Monday everything would close. On the Thursday (a few days prior on the 19th March 2020) something possessed me to write this post:

Gratitude turns what we have, into "enough."
..

For you students who always wished you never had to go to school everyday; I told you if it was taken away from you you'd realise how lucky you are in this country to the right of a free education.
..

For those of you who complained about going to work, how is your workplace functioning now? Do you now question your sense of purpose?
..

For you individuals who were never active enough, how do you feel about the possibility of gyms being closed and now you've lost that opportunity, that everyday you wasted and took for granted.
..

For all of us who eat mindlessly and unconsciously, how unnerving it feels going to the supermarket and not having our "basics" available or even rationed, I bet now you've started to think carefully about what you put in your basket and what is necessary or important for your body to consume.
..

For those who complain about their partners, wives and husbands, imagine them not being there anymore due to sickness.
..

I hope some good comes out of this time we are living in. It may even make people realise that we are like the animal kingdom after all and it really is the survival of the fittest!
..

Your body and health should always be a priority and nothing is worth jeopardising that, I learnt the hard way if you read my previous post.
..

For me, training is my life, and to be honest I'm one of those people who never actually thought about it ever being taken away. All I know is, if today was my last day- I'd make it the best deadlift session to date!
..

Always remain grateful and remember: everything we have left will always be "enough".

Things were seriously changing. We hadn't even gone into lockdown yet, but the shops were manic. There was nothing left on the shelves; no toilet roll, no pasta, no bread, no rice. All the basics. There were queues of people a mile long down the streets snaked across car parks. Boxes or lines were spray painted on the ground, intimidating signs saying, "KEEP YOUR DISTANCE." A slight cough or a loud sneeze would cause heads to turn abruptly. People would see you from afar and cross the road to avoid passing. It was ingrained in us to avoid all contact with people. It became a post-apocalyptic world. Strange, surreal. Some workplaces had already shut down and people were working from home for the first time in their lives. That anxiety that was buried deep inside of me was slowly starting to resurrect itself.

We kept asking each other for reassurance; 'Will we have to shut? What are we going to do?' I needed work. I kept thinking; how will I pay my share of the rent? How will I survive mentally without training? I was in such a bad place in 2015 before training, I had no idea what effect it would have on me if I couldn't train at all in a gym. I didn't even want to imagine it. I couldn't return to that dark place I was in, those years previous.

Saturday 21st March 2020. Our busiest day in the gym. Charlotte and I along with others finished our shift up until midday. I kept complaining of my headache, Anton was also ill but we still remained light hearted and as a joke, he hugged one of his clients who said half-jokingly, 'Oi I don't want your Covid' (little did we know a week later he would have it). Charlotte was advising me not to train. But of course, the stubborn person I am, didn't allow anything to get in the way. I got through, even though I just did not feel myself and lived the rest of the weekend as normal.

Sunday 22nd March. We were told of the possibility that we would be following other countries and going into a full lockdown. Monday and Tuesday we worked as normal, and from Wednesday 25th midnight it was formally announced the UK would be in full lockdown.

And it happened. Just like that. The world as we knew it, would never be the same again.

Anton was single at the time and lived alone, so there was no way I was letting him be by himself, with no gyms, no work, not even being allowed to see your friends and family. It was out of the question; he would stay with L and I until all of this was over.

We all sat nervously, wringing our hands, biting our fingernails and leaning over in anticipation to hear what was yet to be announced as Boris Johnson gave his speech on the TV. Death rates were soaring, and we were in complete disbelief as numbers in the thousands flashed across the screen. We couldn't imagine not going to work, not training in the gym, not being allowed to see friends, no freedom whatsoever, every liberation snatched away from us. Everything that makes life worth living was being taken away.

The first two weeks were awful. We felt awful. Napping throughout the day, lazing around because we had no energy and no purpose to our days. Then we completely lost our sense of taste and smell. It was the strangest experience. I remember cutting up garlic and onion and not being able to smell anything. I even put a raw garlic glove in my mouth and still couldn't taste a thing! Chocolate tasted the same as vegetables, vegetables tasted the same as coffee, everything was tasteless. The only thing we could "taste" or feel rather were textures.

Like everyone around the whole, COVID became that time where everyone realised a lot about themselves; what was important to them, how much loneliness can eat away at you, how it can destroy relationships. It certainly made me reassess my life, what I wanted and even on many occasions, made me question my relationship with L. Did I want to be with him as a person, or did I just need him to mask the loneliness of having nothing else?

Our eating was all over the place. We were eating four bowls of cereal a day despite not being able to enjoy the flavours and the worst thing was we couldn't even train. This lasted two weeks. We were using food as a coping mechanism, to deal with dead time and purpose.

At the time, a new app Disney Plus came out, so I was watching between two to four movies a day, filling the void. It was so strange going from such a high output, waking up for 6am clients, being productive and busy to then waking up to nothing and no purpose. No plans, no goals, just staying at home and playing the waiting game for this to pass. No one had any idea how long any of this would last for. In the 2 weeks we fell ill, Anton and I purchased some resistance bands online and trained a few times from home-until we realised that we were both too strong to train in this way and desperately needed dumbbells and barbells. We hated it and a few times said we didn't know how people got a good workout at home.

One of our most hilarious workouts was me trying to goblet squat Gurgi and me jumping on Anton's back so he could squat me. Our little routine consisted of waking up in the morning, doing a HIIT workout of three rounds then breakfast. It was during this time that I mastered the protein pancake, and my Instagram was filled with much pancake spam. We would go for an hour and a half walk everyday-around the park and across the fields and we would talk about everything and anything-life, this lockdown, Anton's love for someone (who's now actually his partner) and we would head back home.

I will never forget how beautiful the weather was during this first lockdown. Every day was 20 degrees or more. Walking the green hills near the park watching the blossoms awaken for spring, feeling the sun's rays on our skin, and observing the golden daffodils grow, was the only real reminder that life in nature continued.

Other than completing Disney Plus, other parts of the day would involve a few afternoon naps and lots of reading. I missed my weekly trips to the library so much that I started buying second handbooks online. By the end of the lockdown, I counted that I had read over fifty books. Time was going more slowly but we were making up our own routine. If it was a food shop day (once a week on a Friday) I would go as only one person from each household was allowed. The queues to enter the shops would sometimes be half an hour maybe more, people spiralling snake-like around the car park.

No one had ever known anything like it. I would get the basics; bagels if we were lucky, meats and vegetables. The basic human right of living in the Western World to walk into a store and have all matter of foods readily available, was something every person now knew we had taken for granted our whole lives. There was rarely any eggs, bread, flour or toilet roll. Cereal and chocolates and other foods of lower nutritional value were plentiful. While I was out, the boys would often play PlayStation and then by the time you knew it, it was dinner time. In the evenings we would binge through Netflix until bed before we started another day. And it continued like this for the next nine weeks.

After 2 weeks of training at home, we secretly started driving to the gym studio to train (as long as no one else was there). It was frightening because on the news, people were getting fined for not staying at home. I was genuinely worried what would happen if I got caught. I had to have some shopping bags on my back seat and prepared myself that if I was stopped by the police, I would lie and say I was getting shopping for my uncle or nan. The thing is, we had no choice. I couldn't live without training; it wasn't just about my physical health, but I was worried what would happen to me mentally if I couldn't train.

It was madness, it felt like I was in some dystopian, post-apocalyptic film. This didn't make any sense to me that it was an offence, completely illegal to do what was good for my health. Yet people were dying, and I felt that although it was necessary to stay at home at the time, I believe there should have been more effort on the government's part to focus on health. Yes, many died with no underlying health conditions but besides the elderly, individuals who were overweight or morbidly obese, diabetic and high blood pressure were very much at risk, especially being a respiratory illness. Forcing these people to stay at home and live a complete sedentary lifestyle was not benefiting them whatsoever.

This carried on, training in secret until lockdown ended towards the end of July, a whole four months later. It was horrible not training clients, not feeling like you had a sense of purpose. We had a couple of online clients but other than that, absolute zilch. I wasn't earning anything, yet we still had to pay for shopping and our regular outgoings. It finally came out that mortgages were allowed to be put on hold for a few months and I felt so thankful for that at least.

The news kept going on about financial help for the self-employed, but I was so disappointed to find out that I wasn't entitled to anything. Firstly, I hadn't been self -employed long enough to be entitled to anything as you needed at least two tax years behind you and secondly, I wasn't even entitled to Universal Credit because they looked at your partner's income and L earned too much for the Government to support me. I learnt to live within my means. I shopped cheaply and only got what was necessary, we weren't paying the mortgage, and I didn't need to top up on petrol as I was only driving to and from training.

My output remained very low though as there wasn't much to do at home so besides walking and training four times a week, I was still eating the same if not more on some days, so my weight continued to increase. I still remember my first weight training session back after having Covid. Oh my god, it was terrible. I felt I couldn't breathe, recovery was bad, and my strength had completely flopped. I was struggling to hit 60kg on a deadlift. But as the weeks and months went by, I was so pleased that at least besides not working, having no income, I had L, we had Anton staying with us for nine weeks which was so fun, and we had training. I was grateful. I had everything I needed. We all knew we would look back on this time and know we lived it to the full, spending this much quality time with each other that no one else may ever live to do again.

Every day that went by, all we heard was negativity on the news and radio. After a few weeks it was getting us down so much that we all decided that as a rule we would not have it on in the house at all and we would only have it on if there was a new update or announcement about when we were going to come back to civilisation. Every Thursday at 8.00 p.m. we would clap for the NHS and it was the only time we would see anyone else from their windows, balconies and gardens, the only signs of real life and existence. It was a strange concept not seeing other people or interacting with them. We were living in our own little bubble.

The number of deaths was continuously increasing, and it was said that they were using ice rinks to store the bodies. Other rumours were going around including a voice recording from someone high up in the NHS that ambulances were not attending calls as they were scarce, and people were dying at home. You just didn't know what to believe or who to believe. You even suspected your own neighbours as many were turning on each other if they'd discovered you were seeing people or suspected you might be having gatherings!

The roads were completely empty, the only positive thing. Fear would snake its way into you and every time I left the house, I felt I was constantly looking over my shoulder. No more than two people at a time were allowed to be seen out together. More rules were being enforced even not going out for more than one hour a day! I couldn't believe it. Well, Gurgi needed the toilet twice a day so there was no way we could only walk him once. I was constantly made to feel like I was doing wrong; I craved my place in the world, to keep my mental health in check and yet, every liberation was taken away. We were prisoners.

I really wanted to be working again and never for a split second ever wished I was teaching again. Looking back now, we really did make the most out of that time. It taught me to appreciate life and freedom even more, it reminded me how much I loved my job, because it had been ripped away from me. I would often look at stage pictures and really want to start prep again. I wanted nothing more than to compete in 2021 and I knew that all of this would be over by then.

Despite training I was still over-eating and my weight kept shooting up-obviously it didn't help that my output just wasn't as high before, but I wasn't willing to sacrifice any more calories! I managed to go from 144lbs in the April lockdown to coming out of lockdown July and August I was my heaviest ever-152lbs on average and at one point showed 155lbs on the scales. I remember Anton saying that this prep was going to be a very long one, just because I would have 35lbs to lose!

A month before the end of the first lockdown (June 2020) I posted my off-season body for the first time with this:

Off Season 2020:

Not my leanest. But I'm the strongest. NOTE: not your average progress pics- check out my little helper.
..
I'm posting pics of my current physique, as I think it's important to keep it real and show that aesthetics are not always a goal. After my shows, my priorities were getting my health back (For example, cycle/ hormones) and to hit some PBs this year.
..
TRUTH: it is so hard not to compare yourself to your stage weight and for me, accepting how I look when 1. You've been at your leanest for

2 shows 2. You work in the fitness industry and there is a pressure to look a certain way and 3. Social media is always in your face portraying women on many occasions in an unrealistic way.
..

Off season updates:
- *My performance is the best its ever been and I've hit some PBs this year on squats, hip thrusts and deadlifts. Now I'm not too far away from my PB goals that I set myself this year!*
- *Maintaining my current weight (bit heavier than my "bulk weight") and may need to get it down before I start prep in October to avoid a longer cutting phase.*
- *No longer obsessing over numbers. Roughly hitting 2000cals and some days a little more, some days less. I'm going by how I feel.*
- *My quads and glutes have grown-this was my focus hence doing 3 leg sessions a week*
- *Since becoming a PT, my form especially in major compounds has improved massively*
- *My cycle is consistent and all hormones functioning as normal. • Post show injuries have gone and I can bench and squat again (butt to floor as opposed to box) after months of eliminating them. Thank you COVID for giving me that long rest to heal!*
- *I understand my body more now than I did in my last off season and know how to fuel for optimum performance.*
..

Note: I'm not saying having a high body fat % is healthy or vital to hit loads of PBs. What I am saying is that for me, although being heavier than I wanted to be post show, I strongly believe I would never have been able to hit those PB numbers being lean. Admittedly, at this stage I'm not someone that has the same body all year round, although that's a goal for the future. Watch out for my next post on my current PB stats!

My mind at that time was anticipation and excitement to start prep, I felt I needed some focus, discipline and a path. I'd accepted my body, but I was certainly not happy with it nor comfortable. I wanted to be lean. I wanted to change, and I wanted to embark on that journey again. I kept thinking about getting back on stage and what it would be like, how I'd feel that fire in the pit of my stomach again. I even envisioned what my bikini would look like; emerald green. It's amazing the things you can imagine and manifest in your head, even to this day I remember my full routine off by heart. I remember all those nights leading up to show day and every night going through it in my head just before I would go to sleep. Struggling to endure those leg sessions with Anton, memories of him saying 'imagine that trophy at the end of the track' to get me through, stained my mind. When you want something so bad, it's so easy to imagine and envision it and you don't even care how long it takes.

By September 2020, I was fed up with feeling this way. I found it hard to avoid putting on weight and what's worse, my weight gain was not stabilising. At times, I genuinely thought about reaching out, contacting a therapist or a food addiction group. Food was in my head relentlessly. I just HATED NOT FEELING FULL. I HATED HAVING A RELATIONSHIP WITH FOOD as opposed to just viewing it like most people, as fuel to survive. I was in desperate need of that detachment from it. I ate until I was full, even if it meant overeating. I recall following Stephanie Buttermore, a woman in fitness with over 600k followers and was astounded by her profile. What made her stand out so much from everyone else in our industry was her approach to getting over her disordered eating, by a two year 'All In' journey. This meant that despite putting on loads of weight, she avoided tracking (being a previous fitness competitor) and ate well and healthily until she was full, in order to correct her hormones. Seeing her realness, despite the negative comments she received about her physique that she was 'fat', she ended up correcting it and after that, dropped loads of weight again in a healthy way. So, I suppose looking back, had I recovered fully from disordered eating? Probably not. I'd say, I was more so doing the 'All In' approach and trying to repress the feelings of unworthiness that came with it, knowing I'd be competing again.

On September 27th, Anton started my second prep again (probably to avoid me gaining any more) but I was excited about it and I felt ready. This meant I would be on a prep for about twenty-seven weeks and I had 35lbs to lose. It was going to be a hard slog, but I was prepared to do whatever it took to look even better on stage this second time around.

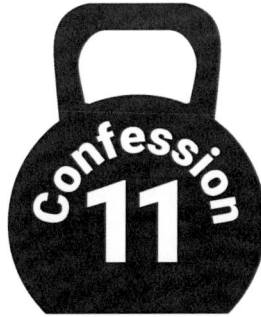

Failure

"Only those who dare to fail greatly can ever achieve greatly."
Robert F. Kennedy

Being on prep this second time round was an absolute breeze. On some days I just couldn't quite believe how easy it was. I wasn't panicking over food, wasn't worried about bulk cooking a week in advance, in fact, I was pretty laid back. Training didn't feel any different. The only things I may have done differently this time round was having a warm, cooked breakfast in the mornings that consisted of a bagel with eggs, smoked salmon and spinach. It certainly filled me up more than baked oats which I had religiously last time. Having a bagel was something I never had in my diet last prep, so you could say I was keeping a wider variety of foods in and avoiding demonisation of foods.

I learnt my lesson last time with my constipation from a lack of fibre, so I was enjoying having half a bag of stir fry veg with my lunch and stir fry broccoli, kale, spinach and peas for dinner. I was always satiated.

Several life changes occurred. Anton left the gym we worked at and where I had trained with him for the first time as his client. I hated not working alongside him and everyone including myself kept saying how the atmosphere just wasn't the same. I hated not being with my best friend every day. It just became such a sad place.

By this time, I was working on two different sites, and it felt lonely a lot of the time, even though I still loved the job and I still had Charlotte. A few times I would meet up with Anton in the Costa close by (he was only working at another gym down the road, so it wasn't too far) but regardless, the job started to become less enjoyable.

I was working A LOT. Many 6.00 a.m. starts and many 9.00 p.m. finishes, sometimes it felt like Groundhog Day.

I missed working with Anton, it just wasn't the same and for about three weeks I was gutted not being together. He left November 2020 and within a couple of months I left too. Taking another leap of faith, I knew my next step was working for myself fully and being in control of my own pay and my own working hours.

Another December came round again, and we were faced with another lockdown. Leading up to this I had developed a reputation and three clients decided to come with me. It turned out that even with just three clients, I was still in a much better position. The gym I was at took a huge cut and I was earning a measly £20 an hour and having to slog long hard hours. Now I loved the liberation I felt. I had fewer clients but working less hours and earning more or less the same. Yes, it was a risky time, but sometimes taking risks are necessary for you to know your worth. Shortly after, Mike and Charlotte followed suit. It was great having full control of my own schedule, own clients and for the first time in my life, not having anyone to answer to or tell me what to do, nor boss me around or treat me like shit.

So, a week before Christmas (2020) lo and behold, good old Boris Johnson lived up to the rumours that were going round, and we were yet again in another lockdown. I couldn't believe it. Shortly before this, I had already met the owner of the gym Anton was at and it was agreed I would start. But this second lockdown ended up lasting another four months! This time I was not willing to sit around on my arse passing the time away, I was going to think of myself and start growing mine and Anton's business. So, although I had a lot of time during the day, clients were mainly done in the morning and Anton, and I would sneak into the studio to train in secret. I was on prep; it was different this time. I had no equipment at home and living in a flat, there was no way I'd be able to squat or deadlift without a bar. I felt so grateful to still be able to train, just as much for my mental health as well as for this prep.

That's not to say I still didn't feel low.

My show dates kept getting moved and it was both a blessing and a curse. A curse because it kept happening (at least twice) so unfortunately prep was lasting longer and longer. At this rate I was going to compete in July. It was a blessing in the sense that it taught me how to maintain my weight. Although my calories were increased I was still having to weigh and calculate everything to a T to ensure I wasn't going over my calories.

Christmas came and it was great. It was the one day I was allowed to eat what I wanted. I had my usual bagel and eggs for breakfast with smoked salmon and spinach and then saved myself room for the big dinner. Despite being banned from socialising at Christmas, I still went round my mum's house. But when I jumped on the scales the next day I was up by 8lbs!!! I was shocked, I didn't even eat until I felt sick or really bloated or full. For those of you who may not have experienced this before, these are the facts. You can't put on fat in one meal. Having been three months in a deficit, believe it or not, the leaner you are, the more prone you are to putting on weight, AND the more prone you are to water retention due to high sodium levels. It was crazy, just one day back on my diet, my weight dropped by 4lbs and the day after another 2lbs so by the end of the week I was back to normal. It was mad: "Each 1 gram of sugar requires 3-4 grams of water to measure and store it." (2020, Wellversed.in/blogs/articles)

I looked good though. I was so focused on building our business I started putting in more effort into my social media with regular posts. I started archiving personal content and switched my account to a business one. My main goal was to start getting myself known, to build my client base.

During the lockdown, an amazing thing happened. Anton who has been affiliated with the company Grenade (they are famous for their protein bars!) invited a guest to come along with him to do some shooting. I couldn't believe it; I was invited for the day!

It was legal because we had to take a Covid test before we went and because it was for advertising and filming purposes, it was allowed. I loved every part of it. We had to travel all the way to King's Gym in London, and I had fluttering butterflies in my belly the whole time. I didn't know what to expect. On arriving, I was so overwhelmed with how amazing the gym looked. It was huge. Every machine you could possibly imagine over two floors.

It also saddened me. It was cold, empty and silent; all the things a gym shouldn't be. We all commented on how sad it was to see an empty gym in this way, it didn't look right at all. We met the CEO of Grenade, the videographers, photographers and the other ladies in charge of the clothing and promotions. I was so surprised when the women there told me to try on the new female apparel for various videos and photoshoots which they would be promoting. I couldn't quite believe it-I was only so happy to be asked, and thankful that I shaved my armpits that morning! It was the most amazing experience of my life (other than competing) just because I had never known this life before.

Anton and I were filmed in a few comedy sketches, and I was asked to have photos taken in the new female apparel with the brand-new energy drinks which tasted amazing! I loved every second. It was the longest day, over five hours in total. (I felt I had a glimpse of an experience of what it must feel like for actors who work long hours, whole days and evenings) but it was so fun.

By the end of the day, I was contacted by the lady in charge, and she informed me she wanted me on board. I was elated.

Me. A part of Grenade, the only protein company I have ever really truly believed in. Plus, I was given £150 in Grenade vouchers for my time that day which I was really happy with. I couldn't wait to do more projects with them.

On the 9th March, Anton and I created a comedy sketch (filmed by L) announcing the news, it was hilarious and we had so much fun doing it. I also wrote this post:

I never believed back in 2015 that completing a training session with @antonkostalas to help my mental health and get me out of bed everyday would have led to now.

Training got me out of the pit of despair I was in. Training led me to compete, training led to my career doing a complete U-tur, training led to working with my best friend everyday and building our own business and training led to this moment and all future ones.

People may not understand why I train. I say: never underestimate the endless possibilities that could come your way or dreams that could be achieved when you do something you love.

So excited to announce being a part of the Grenade team alongside my brother @antonkostalas An amazing brand I have always loved and believed in.

@Grenadeofficial here's to GETTIN' SHIT DONE.

That was their slogan. 86 people liked the post, and I received endless messages of congratulations. I felt like my career was taking off again. My social media was evolving; lots of promotions for Grenade whether it be photos promoting their female attire, their products or funny comedy sketches with Anton and L-it was so fun and didn't even feel like work.

I was even more focused on competing and kept imagining the result. We were still training in secret.

But one day, fear punched me.

Upon arriving and parking across the road from the gym, I observed a police car parked outside the gym and continued to sit there for a good 20 minutes. It was so annoying to think waiting for them to leave was eating into my training time. I thought it even more preposterous that it was illegal to care about your mental and physical wellbeing. Did the government not understand that prioritising your health was helping other vulnerable people? Saving them from taking up another hospital bed? It still astounds me now how priorities are not forthcoming or advised or promoted at all, even though despite the obvious elderly, the other 'vulnerable' who died from Covid were obese, those with diabetes and generally very bad health.

Whereas we were genuinely scared in the first lockdown, this second lockdown only brought more anger and resentment, knowing that the Government cared more about reopening pubs and restaurants before gyms. Their priorities were all wrong and it angered me.

Even though the future seemed bleak, we finally had a date from the government when gyms would be reopening. April 12th 2021. Training in secret, training clients in secret were my daily routine and after that Anton and I would often discuss ideas of what we wanted our future business to look like. We had already planned we would be starting to build our online with a 28 Day Back To Gym Challenge. It was the start of moving forward, a life after Covid.

April 12th came around quickly and admittedly, after 4 months of training in isolation, I felt nervous about my first leg session back. It was strange training with other people around me again, I was excited yet nervous. One thing for sure, it was amazing having machines back in my life again. Doing just compounds and only having dumbbells and barbells can really take its toll on your joints, it felt so nice to have the leg press, extension, curls and hack squats back in my regime.

A couple of months back into routine Anton and I moved gyms again, still close by and although it felt annoying having to start all over again in a new environment after so much change already, we settled in quickly. Rent was better and it meant I had to experience leading classes for the first time, in addition to my own clients.

Show dates were moved again and it turned out the only show date was in July and one show only. I didn't see the point of all that effort for just one show and twenty minutes on stage, so I decided to do the October 2021 shows instead- or so I thought.

Being on a diet for so long was starting to take its toll. I started getting fed up of tracking the same things every day, the shows feeling so far away and my relationship with L was getting harder. We were still so limited with eating out and I was starting to miss 'normal life.' It almost seemed easier during the second lockdown because no one was going out, no one was really socialising. Now that things were getting back to normal, I craved that fun, doing the normal things like eating out, not worrying about weighing everything.

Mentally it was becoming harder, probably because the whole prep felt stop/start and was going on for far too long. Work was getting busier, I was getting a bit more tired but mainly fed up with dieting.

It had been nine months or so and I still didn't even have a period (the only time it had a brief comeback was when I was maintaining my weight for those few occasions of stalling the diet). It was becoming harder and harder to adhere to it. Cravings were high and on a couple of occasions I would slip up and have a slice of bread with jam, then cry afterwards because I'd overeaten by about 200 calories. I recall on one occasion sitting on our balcony and weeping because of it and then crying to L that 'I just want to be normal', yet I knew it wasn't. Stress levels were increasing, and I was starting to question whether I really wanted this and whether it was worth feeling these feelings every single day.

It was a typical spring day in June. Warm and bright, that kind of typical spring day where you start to see the pink and white blossoms awaken to welcome another summer. Everyone appears to have a more relaxed gait compared to the harsh, brisk stances of people trying to shield themselves from the cold and the rain in the winter months. Now, everyone seemed to have a spring in their step again. Everything seems better when it's the warmer part of the year, everyone seems happier. Yet, this day was to be the day that changed everything for me. For me, Anton and my whole family.

Towards the end of a training session with one of my kid clients, I glanced down at my phone; I had received some missed calls from my dad's wife (both who live in Dorset.) I knew immediately something was wrong. It's fair to say that seeing my dad once a year was the best indication of what our relationship was like. Some years it was much less. During the session a text came through; my dad had had a heart attack. Time stood still. I didn't quite know how to feel. I was in so much shock, I waited until the end of my session to call my stepmum.

This day changed everything. For those of you close to me and understand my history; my mum and dad's bitter divorce when I was seventeen, catalysed the breakdown in the relationship with our dad. We had chosen to live with our mum but facing a few years of rejection from our dad affected Anton and I.

At one point in our life, we never heard from my dad for a year and a half. My dad was absent for the biggest most important time of my life growing up. He never knew when I passed my driving test, he wasn't at my graduation, nor did he see me become a teacher or a Head of English. I don't blame him. There were probably a lot of things he was going through mentally. Only now at an adult age do I understand this, and I do not blame him for the breakdown of the relationship. Yet, despite feeling and thinking all of this in that moment, something in me that day changed.

The oddest thing about this whole situation was that we had seen my dad two weekends previously. Since Covid, we hadn't seen him for a very long time, it may have been a year and a half, maybe more.

Anton and I had decided to see him; too much time had gone by. It was on the journey back home after seeing him that weekend, that something made me feel uneasy, anxious and upset. I was unsure at the time whether it was just because it had been such a long time since I'd seen him, but regardless, I felt strange.

At one point on the journey home, I turned to L and I said, 'I'm worried my dad is going to die of a heart attack. He's overweight and his own dad died of a heart attack at this age.' L tried to reassure me that I was maybe feeling a bit down because I knew I wouldn't see him for a while again and also because it was one of the loveliest weekends I've ever had with my dad in my whole life. It felt like we were a normal family. Yet, no more than fourteen days later, it happened, he had three heart attacks with an 80% blockage in one of his arteries. How he survived was an absolute miracle. However, the only thing spinning around in my head was the fact that I had predicted this. It was a feeling that I always refer to as my "magical gut" and it's never wrong. I almost felt as if I was to blame for it, I had jinxed it, I had manifested it and it was all my fault.

The next few weeks were stressful. Anton and I went down to Dorset to see him. It was an emotional rollercoaster, yet we had never felt so close to him; my dad broke down.

I had not ever seen my dad cry since the separation from my mum and it was so painful to see. He then went on to admit to us that he had a serious binge eating problem, that he had suffered with his whole life. I was heartbroken, yet I could relate. I cannot forget his posture as his head fell forward onto his chin, his hands clasped, as his diamond tears rolled round his cheeks and you know that kind of cry when someone struggles to breathe, where their back spasms in line with their breaths. It was one of those painful ones. I broke down and hugged my dad so tight and told him I loved him. My dad could have slipped from my fingers, life really is precious. When we left, I cried and cried. I didn't want to leave him, and I hated that he lived over three hours away.

Over these few weeks, despite being spot on with nutrition and training, my body stopped responding to the diet and was refusing to drop any more weight. On one of the weeks Anton dropped my calories and put in three power walks and my weight still refused to drop. I couldn't believe that my body was reacting in this way from the amount of stress and anxiety I was experiencing: "Stress causes the body to produce more of the hormone cortisol: cortisol is a stress hormone that promotes body fat and makes it harder to lose weight." (Coyle, Motivation Weight Management website)

The weekend we visited my dad, we also went round to my mum's house to watch the football and I broke down in her kitchen. Anton said he hated seeing me like this and it was true. My body was refusing to drop weight, my relationship was becoming strained, I was crying every single day, and I was becoming more and more frustrated with feeling like I wasn't getting anywhere. Anton looked at me and to this day I will never forget his words: 'Tash, I'm telling you as a brother, pull out. As a coach I'm telling you, stop this now.' I was devastated. That night, I knew deep in my heart it was over. Stepping on stage had slipped through my fingers.

That morning, I woke up as normal and I knew that despite paying for the first show, I couldn't go through with it. I sat in the car for about half an hour before my leg session thinking for so long. I had already spoken to Anton for about an hour that morning going through it all and we both agreed it was the right decision. I took two videos of myself, pouring my heart out to no one, all my emotions and feelings about this life-changing decision. Maybe one day I'll have the guts to post them.

Bawling my eyes out, I expressed all feelings of loss and failure, yet again I knew it was the right decision. The way I was feeling about my dad, my weight refusing to drop due to high stress levels, crying every day, for the first time in a long time, I was in a bad place mentally. I was recognising the same behaviours as last time and I knew this time to detect the signs quickly enough to take action and the only way I was going to move forward was to remove myself from this prep.

Shortly after this decision, poor little Gurgi got cancer and had to have an operation. With competing, it's not like a normal lifestyle diet. Your life almost must be completely perfect for you to succeed. You have to have complete tunnel vision for it and even if I kept that focus which I had, your emotional state has to be stable, and my body was just point-blank refusing to drop any more weight.

Everything around me was crashing and burning.

I guess I called this chapter *Failure* because I did fail. I failed at the prep, I failed to reach stage weight, I failed to compete in the shows. On reflection, I am still just as devastated today as I was then about it. I had people say repetitively, 'It's not like you haven't done it before" which is also very true. But this doesn't take away the fact that your confidence is knocked, your self-esteem is low, and the hype of the whole experience is diminished. Even though I'm fully aware I've done it before and placed, to this day I will never know how far I would have got if I did reach that day. The whole experience is one in which you can only ever just re-tell people. I remembered how I excelled as a teacher, rarely failing in anything. Pulling out of these shows was the first time I had truly failed in something, and the unfamiliarity of it was a heavy burden and difficult to accept.

That feeling you get inside of you in the pit of your stomach is indescribable. You can only live it.

Because we are human and we are not immortal and we are imperfect, failure is inevitable in life. I often wonder if humans never failed, what we would all be like as people and whether it would affect the decisions we make. Yes, I failed at this, but my focus changed too. (Well, it was forced to!)

Setting different and realistic goals to replace the old by coming out of this prep, gradually restored my sense of purpose and fulfilment. I wanted to be in a place where I would celebrate small victories to build my confidence again, even though I would still feel the weight of embarrassment when I had to explain to people that I wouldn't be competing again. In all honesty, I was surprised by some of the reactions and felt happy with a sense of validation when I often heard, 'you're doing the right thing'. It made me conclude that growth and success often come through adaptation and resilience.

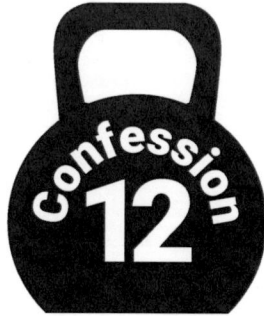

Reverse Dieting

"You don't learn to walk by following rules.
You learn by doing, and by falling over."
Richard Branson

Acceptance is hard with anything, especially for competing. You are forever bombarded with questions like 'are you still competing?' 'When are you next competing?' Not to mention, it is forever on your mind, especially when you're scrolling Instagram or Facebook to observe others who you would have been competing against, seeing their journey, wishing so much it was yours. Once you compete, it's almost like people assume that's all you have been created to do, your only role, your only purpose. The achievement of doing it becomes a defining label, overshadowing any other identity or abilities you could possibly have. People forget the multifaceted person behind the competitor. And competing can cause you to neglect the broader spectrum of who you are and what you could achieve beyond and after it.

One thing I did know after accepting this new situation was even though I felt in limbo, I knew I did not want to be in the same situation as last time where I was binge eating for months on end and feeling terrible about myself. You could say, I was a different me. I was a more positive person; I knew what was to come and I was wanting to learn from past experiences and mistakes.

Hand on heart, this was the best I'd ever come out of a long-term cut. I didn't rush to get my strength back, I ensured to do this gradually and thankfully I didn't get any serious injuries this time. I was more cautious of food and did maintain my weight for a few weeks and still tracked. Unlike before where I went crazy and started eating out a few times a week and binging on rice cakes and other things, I kept to my similar meals, increased the amounts, and limited my eating out to once a week. No, it wasn't perfect, but I still felt proud of myself with how different it felt this time. *I felt different this time.*

It's interesting when a switch or lightbulb moment comes on in your head and you realise your health is more important than anything. More important than looking lean, more important for your mental health, for the female cycle, for everyday life. I did an experiment to see if it was possible to eat pasta without overeating. I ended up having it every day for a week and my weight ended up dropping. It was so nice introducing foods that I wasn't having on prep. I was surprised that eating 100g of pasta was enough. When I think back to my childhood, having one bowl of pasta was never enough. My taste buds and cravings certainly changed post prep this time round. I didn't end up having potatoes or rice for a very long time (months in fact) and instead I would crave just plain bagels and other bland foods.

I was pleased that although putting on some weight during this process, my daily habits were even better than 2020. It's like anything, practice makes perfect. So, practising these good habits certainly benefited me in the long run. Awareness and being so self-reflective constantly aided this success. I was mindful on another level, the complete opposite to how I was at the end of 2019. Going away for my birthday in August in the past I would use it as an opportunity to binge and eat out every day, consuming cake every afternoon but I found I would focus more on what made me feel good. Instead of cake everyday while we were away, I would just have an afternoon coffee and that was enough. My food choices were much better too. On the night of my birthday, I ate curry for the first time in months and I didn't feel sick or bloated afterwards. It was a big milestone for me. Focusing on my health and just feeling good about myself were my main goals.

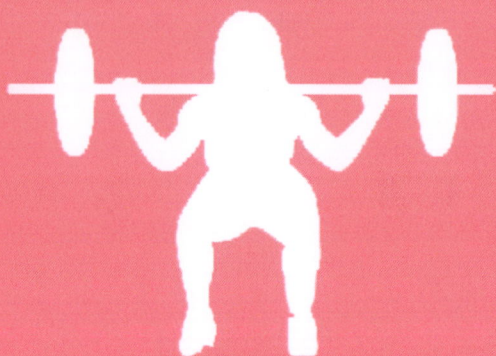

It's interesting when
a switch or lightbulb
moment comes on
in your head and you
realise your health
is more important
than anything.

Even after taking a long break from tracking, I experienced for a few weeks tracking for health, not for a cut. I put myself on 1988 calories; and realised that it was definitely enough food.

In terms of training, I admit I started to feel a little bit demotivated. I never got lazy, but a bit complacent and a little bit bored, I guess. For about nine weeks after this I changed my training for the first time in 6 years. I moved away from the bodybuilding style of training and experienced for the first time a quad and glute programme that Charlotte had done which was VERY different. Everything was high volume (4 sets of 12 squats, 4 sets of 12 hip thrusts, RDLs etc). Even the accessories were high reps like 12 reps at 4 sets of step-ups and kickbacks. I admit I found it quite hard. It was a very strange concept to have to go lighter with weights but have such a great volume. I did it for about 9 weeks in total and missed strength way too much so reverted back to my old way of training. I am really glad I tried something different. It was what I needed after the repetition of training for a show, but also made me realise how much I get the greatest satisfaction out of training for maximum strength and hitting PBs.

My future was unknown, my goals were unknown. During this time for the first time in a long time, there were no goals, and I had no direction. This was my experimental period. A life after competing. I knew that I would carry on working, carry on with good habits, carry on with training, until I knew what I truly wanted.

My future was unknown, my goals were unknown. During this time for the first time in a long time, there were no goals, and I had no direction.

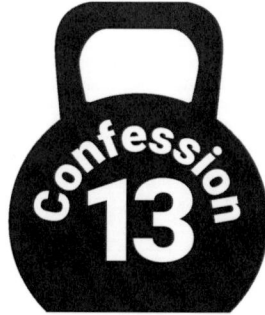

The Anniversary -26/10/2021

'Life is fluid. We are the ghosts of all the people we might become, peering forward to catch a glimpse of what could be, our future selves staring back at us, at who we might have been, never were.'
Bernie Mcgill

I sat in Cafe Nero on North Finchley High Road, London, on the very week I was supposed to have competed again. An oat flat-white coffee on the table and my laptop open in front of me, I began to write; a stream of consciousness. The familiar hum of the cafe provided a comforting backdrop as words flowed as freely as water bubbling in a stream. My reflections and emotions on such a significant day blended the past into the present; a vivid tapestry of thoughts. And this is exactly what I wrote:

I feel strange. Two days ago, would have been the day I would have competed. It's hard to accept that it didn't happen, even though deep down I know it was the right decision. I scrolled on Instagram and saw a few people who won trophies, their excited faces beaming at the camera and even now I sit and wonder what could have been.

Would I have won a trophy?

Would I have placed?

Would I have won a Pro Card?

Would I have been disappointed?

How would that day have gone?

Do I feel jealousy? Envy?

To be honest, I tried to avoid IG as much as possible that day, it heightened my level of devastation. My thoughts creeping, weaving a spiderweb of thoughts. L and I had a lovely day in London that day, but it remained in my mind the whole time we were ambling the streets of London.

In all honesty I feel like my job is not yet done. I keep swaying between competing in powerlifting or bodybuilding because as much as I love training, it's hard keeping motivation high all the time when there is no end goal to work towards. I almost feel like I'm just training to maintain my current weight, training for the sake of training, just a habitual part of my day.

Lately a few people over IG and at the gym have asked 'when are you next competing?' I simply reply, 'I have no idea.' Right now, I feel like I can't actually solidly answer affirmatively whether I would or not. I want to because I feel it is unfinished business.

Then a part of me is worried about two things:

1. *Will my body be able to do it again? Or will I become stressed? Will my body refuse to drop more weight?*

2. *How will I be coming out of it again?*

I'm so worried about going through that horrible process of controlling the binge eating and overeating for months and also worried that I don't want to put on weight drastically again. I fear that the most; going through that long process again of getting back to 'normal'-whatever 'normal' means after competing. The reality is, there is no normal.

This morning, I had a 7.00 a.m. session and with a few minutes to spare, what did I end up doing? Going on the sites to see when the

2022 shows were. One April 2nd which is impossible because my mum is getting married that day and the other date is 8th May. I'm unsure what spiked my curiosity but for some reason it hasn't left my head. I also get scared of what will happen to my relationship. Could that potentially be at stake?

I can envision it though. I can envision the bikini I wanted; I can envision my body changing. I can envision the sound of the crowds screaming my name, the lights brightening up my face, creating sparkly reflections off my bikini, the music booming and encapsulating with every graceful step I take across the stage.

But I fear failing. I have even thought that if I were to do it again, I would do it in secret. I wouldn't share it on my story, I wouldn't tell a lot of people, I would simply justify doing a mini cut until I got close enough to the show dates to share it with people.

Could I do it again?

I just feel like I failed before, so is it possible to accomplish again? I even have my photoshoot all booked and ready. When I pulled out the shows, the photographer said we could postpone. I don't know what 2022 may have in store for me but there is a big part of me that wants to do it so much.

As I read over this now, I can see how deeply I craved a goal, with guaranteed success at the end of it. What did I want? Despite the drive I sense in what I've written, I realise I wasn't prioritising my health, but rather reverting back to familiar patterns. Why would I want to experience binge eating again by wanting to compete again? Yes, getting into condition again would be an achievement, but would it be the right thing for me long term? Absolutely not. It's clear that my pursuit of success would overshadow the need to take care of my physical and mental wellbeing, a habit I needed to break. It's clear I was lost. I sense my struggle to find purpose and clarity and sense of direction. I needed to truly find myself. But how? My road was unknown.

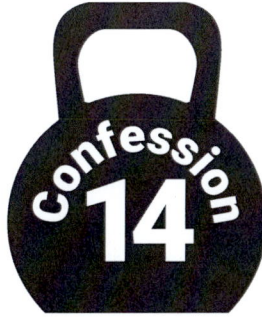

Heartbreak

"Sometimes good things fall apart so better things can fall together."
Marilyn Monroe

When you write a memoir, you often wonder how honest you should be. You are constantly questioning yourself, anxious about how many people will be deeply hurt by what's been written. Hurt by the truth.

I am that individual that writes from the heart and writing the truth has been my main goal throughout this whole process. Writing about the deepest, most personal side of my life outside of my career, outside of my day to day and instead, delving into my inner core, exposing my deepest of feelings is the fairest thing to you.

I am that individual that writes from the heart and writing the truth has been my main goal throughout this whole process.

I truly believe your mind and body go hand in hand. If one is not functioning in the right way, then the other will be affected. Your mind affects your body and your body affects your mind. For example, when you look at an extremely overweight or obese person, most people would be so quick to judge them; it's their laziness, it's their lack of motivation, they don't respect themselves. What people fail to consider is WHY do they lack motivation? WHY do they not respect themselves? There are always deeper reasons for people being a certain way. Whether that is being unhappy with their body, unhappy with their food habits, all leading to even poorer life choices. There are always deeper psychological issues embedded inside someone that determines the lifestyle that they lead.

Heartbreak is the most painful thing you will ever experience that isn't actual death. Fast forward to 2022 and my life changed more drastically than I'd ever known. No one prepares you for heartbreak when you are young. Your parents never warn you about it, no one can tell you how to deal with it, all you can do is live through it and ride every possible emotion, learning for yourself along the way.

I truly believe your mind and body go hand in hand. If one is not functioning in the right way, then the other will be affected. Your mind affects your body and your body affects your mind.

Often, I would look at young people around me; whether it was a group of teenagers ambling across the street in their fresh, neatly pressed uniform, a young teenage couple kissing and holding hands on a park bench overlooking the pond, or even a friendship group of youngsters laughing and flirting on the train. I would often stare at their innocence and think to myself, you have no idea what heartbreaks you are in for in your lifetime. One day it will hit you and your world will feel as if it has crashed on top of you. Yet, without heed or warning, nothing will ever prepare you for what is to come.

I have experienced both types of breakup; the ones that end your life right before your eyes, ripping your heart into pieces and stamping on it in the process and you feel you could die right there and then on the floor. I will never forget the deep, animalistic, loud screams and cries of my very first break up when I was 20 years old. Every object, every song, ANYTHING could be linked back to that person, and you honestly feel at the time that you will NEVER get over this period in your life. Or get over them. No one will ever come close. Your life is over.

Through experience, I have also lived the ones where you must take the initiative. You take on the role of the cruel and heartless one because you are fully aware it is the right thing to do, despite the consequences. This time it was the latter.

L and I were together for five and a half years. I do not regret any decision I've ever made in that relationship, even considering how we came to be in the first place. Love, trust, friendship, we had it all. Yet, for me it wasn't enough. There was always something within me that would make me question my future with him, something that stung me and never really went away for a long time.

One day it will hit you and your world will feel as if it has crashed on top of you. Yet, without heed or warning, nothing will ever prepare you for what is to come.

I repressed these feelings, pushed them aside. I would maintain that relationships change overtime, that everyone becomes settled, comfortable and all that's left to do is carry on. You just stay, that's what people do; it's easier. And that's what I did. But over time, those thoughts crept back in and never really diminished. And everyone knows, when you feel something for long enough, it must be true, they must be real, aren't they?

I guess one of the main issues was I couldn't see us at the stage of having kids and getting married. I know deep down he really wanted children, yet I just couldn't see myself taking on that role, living that life with him.

I maintain if you want something in life and you know the other person cannot or will not give it to you, it's vital you consider your own needs first. I once said to him when discussing this exact topic that if there was something I really wanted in life and I knew for a fact he couldn't give it to me, I would not stay. He loved me that much that he was willing to sacrifice the one thing I couldn't give him in life.

If you want something in life and you know the other person cannot or will not give it to you, it's vital you consider your own needs first.

Some of you may call it selfishness. Life is too short not to live it to the full and fulfil your happiness. You cannot live for someone else; you cannot make someone the only part of your life and you cannot depend on someone to create your happiness or fulfil all your needs. They have to come from within. Your partner should compliment your life, add to it, enrich it, but not be the be all and end all to complete it. That is not healthy. This is how I thought about L and yet wondered why I couldn't be happy with a man who put me on the highest pedestal imaginable, made me his everything, no one riding above in importance.

I don't want to blame competing because it changed my life for the better and led me to who I am today. But, as I have had so long to reflect on my breakup with L, I am fully aware now that competing really did change it forever. It just wasn't the same after that. But that's what happens when you achieve something so difficult and so amazing, you change as a person. Or rather, develop and become a more rounded individual. That person is staring back at you in the mirror, confused as to how you could have altered this much.

When L and I first met, we were just two very vulnerable people that found each other at the right time. We needed each other. He was the lonely, vulnerable man in an unhappy marriage, and I was the unconfident, vulnerable unhappy woman in my career. We both craved an escape out of our situations, and we helped each other to do that eventually. We were seeking solace in each other. We fixed each other.

You cannot live for someone else; you cannot make someone the only part of your life and you cannot depend on someone to create your happiness or fulfil all your needs. They have to come from within.

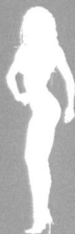

People change and it's not necessarily a bad thing. Without change, there's no growth, without change there is no personal development, without change there is no learning from mistakes or lessons, without change there's no opportunity for reflection. I am a different person from my twenties to my thirties. Undoubtedly, I will be a different person from now in my thirties into my forties. Change is inevitable. You either grow with that person, or you don't. And we grew apart. Because of me.

Knowing you have inflicted this much pain on someone is the hardest thing to live with. All you have in your head are feelings of guilt. I will never get out of my head how he felt, his reaction and knowing I was the one responsible for all of this. Nevertheless, I knew it was the right thing and I hope one day he realises this too. Inevitably, there will be imbalances in relationships, but too many of them will always lead to one in the relationship feeling resentment or unfulfillment.

Knowing you are on your own is the scariest thing to contemplate when you end a relationship. The fear of the unknown. You must accept your new routine, coming home to an empty flat, cooking meals for one. But, making the most of liberation, feeling content with your life and accepting the choice you made was the right one helps a lot. There were times, when I was completely by myself, where for a split second I would have to tell myself this was real, that this really happened, that he didn't exist in my life anymore. During the aftermath, when a negative thought slyly entered my head, I would pull it out aggressively and remind myself of all the positive reasons why I chose this.

Without change, there's no growth, without change there is no personal development, without change there is no learning from mistakes or lessons, without change there's no opportunity for reflection.

There is a big difference between genuine happiness and contentment. I was content with L, but I was not one hundred percent happy with him. I truly believe he was also just content. Was he genuinely happy with me? Was he also subconsciously repressing the same thoughts that I had?

During this time after I ended my relationship with L, training really did take me out of the darkest of times. Training for me now has been the light at the end of the tunnel and the last piece of string that I have clutched on to, forcing me to carry on and move forward. I think it's vital that people never undermine the power of mental strength and what seems an unreachable amount of strength that is able to be instilled within, from something like lifting.

I dropped about 10lbs in one month after my breakup with L. The weirdest thing was, after all this time of trying to drop, I couldn't believe how easy it was. My appetite became non-existent, and I would often have to force feed myself knowing I was training. I was no longer relying on food emotionally. I seemed to do that a lot in the last year that I was with him, seeking comfort in it.

What haunts me the most is the day I told him. It was a normal day in August, we'd just got back from a romantic holiday in Kefalonia, yet my thoughts of ending the relationship had been pervading my mind for weeks, the seed had been planted two years prior.

Never undermine the power of mental strength and what seems an unreachable amount of strength that is able to be instilled within, from something like lifting.

I had another epiphany on this day. I went to work as normal. Came home as normal. And did it. I told him everything. Sat him down and explained I hadn't been happy, and I wanted this relationship to end. That I'd changed and it was what I wanted. As relieved as I was that it had been done, it still plagues my mind, even to this very day. His tears, his breakdown, his shock; his complete and utter disbelief. The person you loved and lived with for years, who meant *everything* in your world, now fades into nothingness. It's like they have died.

The truth is, I felt I filtered so much of who I was when I was with him. I wasn't the real me.

Now, I can live.
Now, I can be the real me.

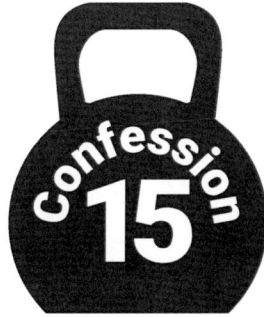

Where I Stand Now

"If you hear or read stories on how successful people achieve their extraordinary accomplishments, most of them always start by stating their secret: they follow their passion."
John Baskin

I often question myself: if I hadn't competed would I still be a teacher now?

Would I have ever had the confidence to close the door of just over a decade of my life? We shall never know.

Would I have had the bravery instilled in me to end my relationship with L? Who knows.

If I never competed, I probably would still be allowing people to abstain a copious amount of blood out of me. I may well be living everyday discontented and unhappy in a job that just wasn't the *real me*, coasting leisurely year after year, complaining relentlessly but avoiding any action of change.

I may have stayed in a relationship I was unhappy in, simply because it was easier. Undoubtedly, *because* of competing, I have a limitless amount of physical and mental strength. And it was solely these two facets that determined every decision I ever made hereafter.

I love working in the fitness industry and I wouldn't change it for the world. But the fitness industry is a complicated one. The fitness world and everything associated with it such as promotions, social media, Instagram girls, half naked individuals with perfect physiques and everything else not aforesaid is equally confounded. On the surface, it is incredibly superficial, there is only so much of a story you can tell from observing a picture. It looks highly glamorised and every individual in it may come across as arrogant, again superficial with perfectly chiselled bodies and perfect lives. But this is only one side.

Competing on the surface, like social media is a counterfeit. Once you peel away the layers, there is just a hollow emptiness. Feeling this way but embracing the challenge associated with competing still remains the best thing I ever accomplished, and I will always be proud that I pushed myself and my body to a place I never thought was achievable. I will never exhibit feelings of regret despite the consequences.

When I grow older, I will look back and think, wow *I did that*. I did what a small percentage of the population can do. Yes, it came with its sacrifices, setbacks, disappointments, effects on my mental and physical health and relationship. But without it, I would not be who I am, who I *really* am, who I have become as a person, *my identity*. It transformed me, yet I will always view me as the same humble person I always was and am. It didn't make me better than anyone else, it just made me a better version of me and made me open my eyes to what is important, especially when I pulled out the second time around.

Yes, deep down I honestly feel I will never have that perfect relationship with food, but with every year that has gone by, I'm learning more and more and developing the lifestyle I want.

I wake up every morning and never once have I associated feelings of trepidation with going to work. It does not feel like a job at all and many in the industry will tell you that too. I don't have the Sunday night blues which I had continually every week for ten years. I wake up, even if it is 4.45am and it's dark and cold with just the patina of the moon guiding my steps as I walk with a coffee attached to my hand and I embrace the fact that I am healthy, I eat well, train well and I love what I do.

I always think to myself I am so lucky to be able to walk, I don't have a serious illness and life really is precious and we must look after our bodies. They are our temples, and we should worship them. I am trying to set myself up to put myself in the best position so that when I become old, frail, and grey I know I did everything I could to be alive, stay alive for as long as possible.

Competing still remains the best thing I ever accomplished, and I will always be proud that I pushed myself and my body to a place I never thought was achievable.

In terms of body confidence and how I view my body, I recall a post I wrote in September 2020 a week before I started my second prep and I wrote a list of all the comments that have been made to me (directly and indirectly) since I started training:

"You're too skinny"

You're big"

"Dench"

"Your face looks gaunt"

"Stacked"

"What's happened to your face?" (Whilst trying to pinch what was left of my cheeks)

"Muscly"

"Shredded"

"You look amazing"

"You're not obese, you just look muscular"

"Tiny"

"Your arms are big, do you go to the gym?"

"You have the best upper body I've seen on any woman in 6 years"

"Strong"

In a conversation about taking steroids "Ohhh you're natural? I thought you took drugs." -(HILARIOUS!)

I recall another moment where a man who passed me by in the street looked me up and down repeating "no, no" and nodding his head in disapproval making me feel inadequate.
..
A bunch of guys in a car as I was walking down the street shouting out the window "how was the gym?" (+loud laughter)

Etc., etc., the list is endless.
..
I have come to the realisation that it's no surprise that I have had that many contrasting comments (both positive and negative) about my body in the last few years. I have been off season, doing a minicut, off season again, prepping for a show or now currently off season again.
..
It's made me realise that although I'm very excited to start prep again in a week's time for my next shows, my next goal afterwards will be the art of maintenance, a whole new challenge for me.
..
If you are someone who is muscle building right now, especially if you're a woman and you don't feel that comfortable with how you look, don't allow negative comments or behaviours to put you off.

Just remind yourself- your end result will depend on how much you've invested and built in your offseason. #trusttheprocess #offseasongains #strongerbodystrongermind

It is no surprise that everyone will always have an opinion of what you look like; competing is all about the Judges' opinions! People comment when you lose weight, but not so much when you put it on!

A month into my second prep in October 2020, I wrote an IG post that really sums up competing:

A year ago today and what have I learnt?

When you do something that challenges you, out of the ordinary or something you thought you never could do, you feel you can do anything.
..
To stop stressing about the little things. Stress from my previous job took over my overall health/ mental health and I will never let that happen ever again
..
Take risks-I always feared change and so would always play it safe. Now I'm finally in a job where I know who I am and doing what I love every day that it doesn't feel like working at all.
..
That doing shows are just the icing on the cake and competing again is for the love of the challenge and all the work and passion I put into the training
..
Never to forget the endless support from people who help you achieve your dreams (especially @el_hembo
..
Everything I've learnt about training, nutrition, passion and having dreams and accomplishing them is because of my brother, best friend and coach @antonkostalas who without him, I would never be who I am today.

To this day I still don't understand why this hasn't changed over the years. I almost think there should be some sort of aftercare for competitors that's included in the price for entering the shows, like a rehab or a session where competitors can discuss disordered eating, body confidence and life after competing. They don't call them post show blues for no reason; many competitors post show experience depression. I wrote a post on this in November 2020:

Post show blues? Here's what you need to know...

- *Don't beat yourself up too much with the binging-your hormones are fudged and you can't process when you're full. This takes time to resolve itself so be patient.*

- *Try and follow macros for 3-4 days out of the week and give yourself a calorie range*

- *Don't obsess too much over numbers-this includes your bodyweight and comparing yourself to your stage weight. Stop weighing out foods to a T like you would normally do on prep like veg and ketchup!*

- *Set yourself new goals. People can feel down because they think once it's done, there's nothing else. Setting myself performance goals (kgs I wanted to hit in my compound lifts) for the year helped me stay focused.*

- *Try and repress negative feelings of worthiness. Admittedly, when I put on more weight than I wanted you almost question whether you are "worthy" enough to be in the fitness industry and confidence is at an all-time low. This goes away with time and acceptance that stage weight is not healthy.*

- *Focus on getting your hormones back to normal. Ladies, if your cycle stopped really focus on getting it back, for example, higher calories and eating plenty of good fats. DON'T stress about your aesthetics.*

- *I would never recommend competing again straight away. I am glad I took 10 months out to get my body back to functioning normally. Your body has been under great stress.*

- *Don't go ham in the gym. I ended up wanting my strength back too quickly and developed injuries.*

- *There is always a next time. You only ever really know that you want to compete again, when you've done the process of coming out of it. I believe it is the greatest most amazing experience, hence why I'm doing it again—roll on April 2021!*

It's incredibly strange to think that I am writing this chapter exactly a year to the day. I do get a bit sad as I read it, especially the last bullet point and think this year could have been my year, but it just wasn't meant to be. I honestly do not know whether I ever will compete again. The most important thing for me is knowing I will always have training. It still excites me, fulfils me and challenges me just as much as the first day I started in 2015.

I wrote a post about that too:

Life lessons that weight training taught me:

Strength, mental strength: dealing with my emotions and stress. When things happen that test you, you realise the pain of squatting feels so much more painful than what's on your mind!
..
Being true to yourself: I remember feeling very lost about 5 years ago when I was still in teaching and I now know who I am and what I want in life.
..
Surround yourself with people that you can learn from: I certainly have—from people modelling what it means to be a fantastic PT, to inspiring me overall as people
..
Learning from mistakes: no stress compares to how I felt in my previous career and I vowed to myself I would never feel an ounce

of that again and if I did, to actually do something about it. It took me a long time to realise that "being selfish" is actually "self-love" or "selflessness" and your own happiness is the most important thing, no matter what anyone else thinks or tells you.
..

Boldness: 5 years ago, I was a "people pleaser" and I remember my Mum once telling me I would grow out of being too nice. I would often do what people expected me to do even when I didn't agree with it or didn't want to. The pressures of being in any matter of constrainment cause relentless acceptance. Saying the truth and speaking my mind reminds me of who I am as a person
..

Liberation: pushing yourself beyond limits in training or training towards something like my shows (what I thought was impossible) reminds me in life that possibilities are endless, and you should never be content with limitations.
..

What life lessons have you learnt through any form of training?

I reflect on my life now and I am in the best job, working with the best clients, growing a business, writing blogs, writing this book, (well written this book if you're reading it!) working with Grenade, can say I have done a podcast and am still able to train kids which was always the best part of teaching. I feel genuinely fulfilled, and excited for whatever the next few years may have in store.

After bodybuilding, I decided I needed a new goal and in April 2024, I "found myself" again and competed in my first powerlifting competition, coming second out of fourteen women in my category. Funny to think I did better in this non-aesthetic sport than I ever did in bodybuilding. I'm now looking to compete in more competitions in the future. We will see where life takes me. Wherever it does, it is due to my relentless drive to keep developing and setting goals. By constantly striving for improvement, I ensure my journey is always purposeful. You never know the window of opportunities that will present themselves.

Since my competing year in 2019, every year I have focused on *me*. My self-development is infinite. I even underwent therapy as another facet of self-development for over six months. Therapy probably isn't for everyone, but for me, I continued to notice the benefits and realisations long after I stopped. Since competing, and through everything I've learnt about myself, I now have clarity on what I want in a relationship, what behaviours I accept from people and which I don't. I know the people I want to surround myself with, and whether they have a positive impact on my life. My journey, following on from competing, has not only improved my physical and emotional wellbeing but also empowered me to set healthier boundaries and make more fulfilling connections.

I'm in the best relationship *with myself*. I have learnt to train for health, train for my powerlifting goals (maybe there will be a sequel: *Beyond the Barbell: Confessions of a Female Powerlifter)*, eat for health and have even experimented with dieting WITHOUT following macros; I managed to lose 12lbs over a period of time. For a long time after competing, I never believed I'd be able to diet again. I truly believed I'd never be able to find food freedom. But I did. And you will too.

If you still struggle with your relationship with food or even yourself, including your body image, remember the following nuggets that I stand by to this day. These small things I look back on, over the last eight years of my fitness career, have transformed my life to such a degree, that I almost wish someone had told me these very things earlier on, instead of learning them through trial and error and working them out for myself:

- *Wear clothes that actually fit you—don't beat yourself up every time you attempt to fit into those pair of jeans—even if temporary, buy nice clothes that fit your body size now.*

- *Don't scroll or follow people on social media that make you feel bad about yourself; only compare yourself to yourself. Remember, you can change your body into whatever you want it to be, but it will always be the best version of what your body could be. This includes only surrounding yourself with positive people who have a good impact on your life.*

- *Don't focus just on body weight: to avoid becoming obsessive, weigh yourself two or three times a week and use other measures of success other than a number on the scales. For example: progress photos, do my clothes fit? Do I feel confident about myself?*

- *Do things that require self-love: whether that be getting your nails done or indulging in a massage. Have a list of things that make you feel good and do them.*

- *Move away from perfection and remember it doesn't exist. You might admire someone and assume they are the epitome of perfection, but they're not. Even in their own heads, they know they are not.*

- *Focus on things you like about yourself. Write a list and when you have a down day, refer to that list. Make sure you put physical aspects on there!*

- *Accept compliments and avoid deflecting, just say, 'thank you'.*

- *Focus on things beyond aesthetics—go to the gym even if it is just for your mental health or focus just on strength. Maybe shift your focus away from 'I want to lose weight.'*

- *Focus on foods that make you feel good.*

Competing is not the be all and end all. It simply opens opportunities because of newly found confidence that becomes *you*. I recall a Martin Luther King quote: "You don't have to see the whole staircase to take the first step" and I guess competing was quite a big chunk of this staircase!

I hope you have felt you have really got to know me through reading my journey. Please learn from my mistakes. Please don't waste days, weeks, months and even years being unhappy and lying to yourself that you are. Whether that's a relationship you feel you're stuck in, a highly paid job that keeps you in your place because you feel there is nothing better, a boss that doesn't know your worth. You don't need to compete to learn from my experience. The only important person is you.

I recall a Martin Luther King quote: "You don't have to see the whole staircase to take the first step" and I guess competing was quite a big chunk of this staircase!

Where do I see myself today and onwards? Well, it's almost like this last part is my own eulogy to myself: I want to be remembered as the female competitor that spoke out. Told you the truth about everything that surrounds competing and being in the world of fitness. I may want to go back into schools one day and help teenagers understand disordered eating, living a healthy lifestyle, learning about how to gain body confidence.

I may compete again, I may not.

I may become a well-known author, I may not. All I do know is I want to stay happy. I now realise if I ever return to that dark place before I started training, I will have the confidence to do something about it.

You don't need to compete to learn from my experience. The only important person is *you*.

Once I thought a number on the scales would keep me happy, that it meant having visible abs, that competing was the only thing that gave me confidence. I truly believe true happiness is feeling confident in yourself, knowing who you really are and accepting that person, accepting your body. Spending quality time with people you love, especially since the life we all led during Covid 19, since I nearly lost my father. Being more relaxed with food, moving away from these guilt cycles has been hard to adapt to after such a long prep without even being able to complete the shows.

I truly believe true happiness is feeling confident in yourself, knowing who you really are and accepting that person, accepting your body.

But life really is too short and too precious and keeping your mental health in check is the rock holding up the rest of your life.

Take leaps, take risks. Because what you may once have believed to be a failure or a huge risk, may be a success in disguise. Your journey will never be the same as everyone else's but own it.

Your mental health in check is the rock holding up the rest of your life.

One thing I do know for sure, I can be ANYTHING I want to be. YOU can be ANYTHING you want to be.

Author's Note

If you're reading this, you reached the end of 'Beyond The Barbell: Confessions of a Female Fitness Competitor.' I hope by reading about my experiences you have learnt something. If anything, you have read here has inflicted any kind of emotion inside of you, then I have achieved my purpose. To enlighten and move you by revealing my truths was my sole purpose for writing the book.

It was always on my bucket list to be a writer and the fact that I can now tick it off has been just as much an achievement as stepping on that stage was, in 2019.

I hope it has taught you that bodybuilding as much as it should be admired, comes with a precaution. If after reading this piece, it is still something you'd like to pursue, then good luck—I have outlined everything you need to know, and I admire your drive and determination. Fundamentally, I wanted to tell my story so you would know that there is more to bodybuilding than the 'perfect' physique. In fact, there is no such thing as perfection.

I hope it has taught you that you never know what is truly going on in someone's life, especially people in fitness and what you scroll on Instagram every single day; looks are deceiving after all. Lastly, I wanted to be remembered as that one person in fitness that spoke out, that says it as it is, reveals all the truths, all the taboos, no matter how hard some chapters were for me to write, some details I have never actually revealed until now.

I hope it has reminded you to thank your body every single day. Accept and nurture it, no matter the size or shape, it's what keeps you going. Make it a promise to keep it strong every single day, for as long as you're living, it will thank you for it.

I'd love to know what you thought about "Beyond The Barbell." Please connect with me on Instagram @natashakostalas and tag me your thoughts.

I am truly grateful to you for reading my story.

Tash x

Bibliography

Abelsson, A. (2022) 'The 10 Best Bodybuilding Splits: a Complete Guide' Available at: https://www.strengthlog.com/bodybuilding-split/#upper-lower-body-split

Anderson, J. Drake, C. Kalmbach, D. (2018) 'The Impact of Stress on Sleep: Pathogenic sleep reactivity as a vulnerability to insomnia and circadian disorders,' Available at: https://www.ncbi.nlm.nih.gov/pmc/articles/PMC7045300/

Andrews, M. (2006) 'Why do Veins Pop out when Exercising, and is that Good or Bad?' Available at: https://www.scientificamerican.com/article/why-do-veins-pop-out-when/#:~:text=This%20process%2C%20known%20as%20filtration,persons%20with%20less%20subcutaneous%20fat.

Bourgeois, C. Forbes Health (2024) 'Reverse Dieting: What to Know' Available at: https://www.forbes.com/health/nutrition/diet/reverse-dieting/#:~:text=Reverse%20dieting%20is%20a%20post,weight%20gain%20after%20a%20competition.

Better Health (2019) 'Menstruation-amenorrhea Available at: https://www.betterhealth.vic.gov.au/health/conditionsandtreatments/menstruation-amenorrhoea#bhc-content

Blogs. Brighton. (posted May 10 2022) 'Nutrition of a peak week for a novice bodybuilder' Available at: https://blogs.brighton.ac.uk/peakweek/#:~:text=During%20the%20first%203%20days,the%20amount%20of%20fat%20consumed.

Boutot, M. (2016) 'Stress and the Menstrual Cycle' Available at: https://helloclue.com/articles/cycle-a-z/stress-your-period

Brigham Health Hub. Robinson and Andromalos (2020) 'Sleep More to eat less: How Sleep Affects the Hunger Hormone' Available at: https://brighamhealthhub.org/controlling-the-hunger-hormone/#:~:text=Research%20has%20shown%20that%20 sleep,sure%20to%20get%20enough%20sleep.

Burke, P. Stets, J. (2014) 'Self-Esteem and Identities' from Sage Journals volume 57 issue 4 Available at: https://journals.sagepub. com/doi/10.1177/0731121414536141

Chappell, A. (2022) ProPrep 'What they don't tell you about contest prep and what to expect' Available at: https://proprepcoaching.com/ science-of-bodybuilding/what-they-dont-tell-you-about-contest-prep-what-to-expect/

Cooley, C. (1902) 'Perception is reality: The Looking-Glass Self', Lesley University. Available at: https://lesley.edu/article/perception-is-reality-the-looking-glass-self#:~:text=The%20looking%2Dglass%20self%20 describes,worth%2C%20values%2C%20and%20behavor

Coyle, M. (2019) 'How Stress Prevents Weight Loss and 3 Ways to Beat it' Available at: https://motivation.ie/stress-management/how-stress-prevents-weight-loss-and-5-ways-to-beat-it/

Cusack, A. Ely, A. (2015) 'The Binge and the Brain' Available at: https:// www.ncbi.nlm.nih.gov/pmc/articles/PMC4919948/

Davidson, K. Mandell, A. Fagan, J. (2017) 'Bodybuilders Develop Binge Eating Disorders Post Competition: A Survey' Available at: file:///C:/ Users/NKost/Downloads/rutgers-lib-51572_PDF-1.pdf

Evans, W. Frank, L. Lambert, C. (2004) 'Macronutrient Considerations for the sport of Bodybuilding' Available at: https://pubmed.ncbi.nlm. nih.gov/15107010/ on off season

Fazackerley, A. (2022) The Observer '90% of schools in England will run out of money next year, heads warn' Available at: https://www. google.com/amp/s/amp.theguardian.com/education/2022/oct/22/ exclusive-90-of-uk-schools-will-go-bust-next-year-heads-warn

Harris, M. (2020) 'Get Poised' Available at: https://www.getpoised.net/post-show-blues-body-image-self-talk-depression-bodybuilding-competition/ explains hormone and depression

Harris, R. (2023) 'Dealing with Post-Competition Depression As Bodybuilders' Available at: https://www.muscletech.com/blogs/journal/post-competition-depression

Harrison, J. (2022) '44% of state school teachers plan to quit by 2027' Available at: https://www.ier.org.uk/news/44-of-state-school-teachers-plan-to-quit-by-2027/

Healy, J. Lee, J. (2011) 'Delayed Onset Muscle Soreness' Available at: https://www.sciencedirect.com/topics/neuroscience/delayed-onset-muscle-soreness#:~:text=DOMS%20is%20described%20as%20muscle,contractions)%20in%20an%20athlete's%20training.

Hunkemoller. 'Gym-Anxiety: how common is it, and how do we combat it?' Available at: https://www.hunkemoller.co.uk/gym-anxiety#:~:text=According%20to%20our%20study%20over,intimidated%20by%20public%20workout%20spaces.

Kluck, A. (2010) 'Family Influence on disordered eating: The role of body image dissatisfaction' Body Image Volume 7 Issue 1 pages 8-14 Available at: https://www.sciencedirect.com/science/article/abs/pii/S1740144509001016

Magwaza, P. (2017) You Magazine Online 'My libido vanished'-bodybuilder choose perfect body over sex' Available at: https://www.news24.com/you/wellness/my-libidos-vanished-bodybuilder-chooses-perfect-body-over-sex-20171018

Marcin, A. (2016) 'Binge Eating Disorder History: A Timeline' Available at: https://www.healthline.com/health/eating-disorders/binge-eating-disorder-history

Mayo Clinic Staff, (May 4, 2018) 'Panic Attacks and Panic Disorder' Available at: https://www.mayoclinic.org/diseases-conditions/panic-attacks/symptoms-causes/syc-20376021

NHS Inform. (last updated 3 June 2024) 'Motor neurone Disease' Available at: https://www.nhsinform.scot/illnesses-and-conditions/brain-nerves-and-spinal-cord/motor-neurone-disease-mnd#:~:text=Motor%20neurone%20disease%2C%20also%20 known,walking

Pacheco, D. Singh, A. Sleep Foundation. (2020) 'Lack of Sleep may increase Calorie Consumption' Available at: https://www. sleepfoundation.org/sleep-deprivation/lack-sleep-may-increase-calorie-consumption#:~:text=Likewise%2C%20lack%20of%20 sleep%20can,to%20a%20higher%20calorie%20intake

Suni, E. (2022 updated April 18, 2024) 'Sleep Paralysis: Symptoms, Causes and treatment,' Available at: https://www.sleepfoundation. org/parasomnias/sleep-paralysis

Acknowledgements

This still doesn't seem real. Writing a book was always on my bucket list and now it is time to tick it off. There are far too many people to thank for this piece getting published, so I will try my best to keep it brief.

Mum: you instilled in me a love of English Literature, a world of writing, culture and of books. Thank you for supporting me in my monumental life changing decision to move away from a world of teaching and into one surrounded by dumbbells and barbells. Without you, I wouldn't have shared that love of reading and literature. I still remember our weekly trips to the library at ten years of age, the nightly reads before bed (even if you fell asleep), the shelving space I needed for my paperbacks, for supporting me through my English teaching career and for sharing my excitement of writing this, something I said you should always accomplish yourself.

My best friend Sam, you officially are my oldest friend. With over twelve years of friendship, I hope you can forgive me for not telling you I was doing this, I wanted it to be a surprise. Thank you for always being there for me, through every milestone that has been my life.

My other beautiful friends Nadia and Polson—I still remember that night at Caminos many years ago. You both pushed me to compete, so nearly all of this is down to you. Thank you for believing in me and shouting at the tops of your lungs on that day in 2019.

All my other TTA friends and Oasis, friends who were there to support me on the day—you all know who you are.

My family for putting up with me. For accepting my funny ways and irritating food habits.

My editor and literary agent, Soulla Christodoulou for being such an amazing friend and mentor during this whole process. You inspire me every day and instilled the belief in me that I could really do this.

L for the time we were together, you accepted me whatever size I was, and whatever avenue I ever walked down, holding my hand the whole way. I hope you find your true love in life.

To every person I have encountered in the gym: for every conversation I've had with you, thank you for inspiring and motivating me just that little bit more.

Last but never least, my brother Anton: my sibling shredder, sibling gainer, coach, teacher, mentor, business partner, partner in crime, confidante, idol, superhero, champion, best friend, brother. How empty my world would be without you. I will never forget your words: 'Tash, you need to start prioritising yourself.' For this, bro, I am living proof, because of you. You trusted and believed in me, always aiding my growth. You embedded and instilled in me a permanent true love of training.

About The Author

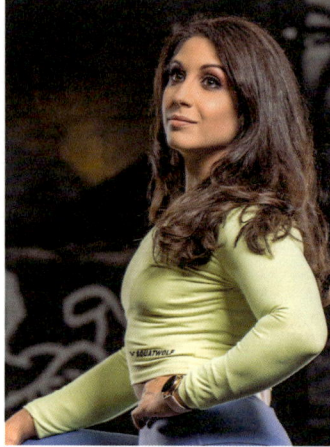

Natasha Kostalas is a former Head of English and English teacher of 10 years turned Personal Trainer after she competed in bodybuilding in 2019. When her mental health took its toll in 2015/2016 due to a toxic relationship and a high-flying role that she abhorred, her road to healing was when she started weight training with her coach and brother, Anton, who was her main inspiration. His positivity and love of weight training inspired her to become better, to become a more positive person and her life was completely transformed thereafter. Watching him compete in bodybuilding only sparked her drive to take her training to the next level and Anton coached her to compete in 2 shows in 2019; she came 5th and 4th in 2 categories.

When Natasha wanted to compete again in 2021, she had to pull out of the shows due to personal circumstances which is what led her to start writing her memoir *Beyond the Barbell: Confessions of a Female Fitness Competitor*. Since then, she's still growing her PT business, has recently competed in the sport of powerlifting, coming 2nd place out of 14 women in her category, hosts her weekly podcast *The Binges to Barbells Podcast* and writes weekly fitness articles on Substack. She is currently working on her second book.

www.ingramcontent.com/pod-product-compliance
Lightning Source LLC
Chambersburg PA
CBRC101140030426
42334CB00008B/119